Is Gluten Hiding in Your Shampoo?

It was Hiding in Mine!

An **eZ** Gluten-Free Shopping Guide
for Personal Care Products

Marian Z Geringer

eZ Gluten-Free Life

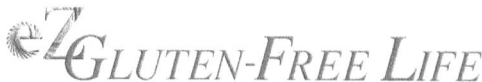

Additional Gluten-Free Handbooks Available:
By Marian Z Geringer

Gluten-Free Living 101
An eZ step by step guide on how to start living a successful gluten-free life today.

Is Gluten Hiding in Your Kid's Things?
An eZ guide: addressing the issues of raising gluten-free children; includes a thorough list of gluten-free products for children and infants..

Marian is currently working on **Is Gluten Hiding in Unexpected Places?**
Gluten can be found in products you may not have considered such as:

Alcoholic Drinks	Fast Foods
Candy	Sauces
Cleaning Products	Spices
Cooking Sprays	and More...

Is Gluten Hiding in Your Shampoo?
It Was Hiding in Mine!
A Personal Care Products Handbook

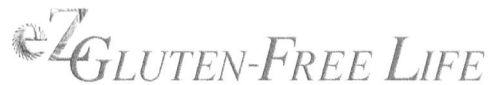
eZ Gluten-Free Life

Is Gluten Hiding in Your Shampoo? It Was Hiding in Mine! Even after I began to heal from my medical issues caused by eating gluten, I continued to have skin issues. As I tried to figure out why the skin rashes and eczema persisted, I discovered that there are over 200 chemical names for ingredients derived from gluten, hiding in body care and personal care products. The process required me to email, call and write to hundreds of personal care product companies to find out which of their many products contained gluten. The process took over 18 months and then had to be repeated in order to confirm the results. As a gluten-free consultant, I continually receive emails and Facebook posts asking me about personal care products. I decided to take all my research and create *"Is Gluten Hiding in Your Shampoo?"* a detailed handbook of gluten-free personal care products.

The handbook is divided into 2 sections.

Section 1: Pages 5 through 14 consist of brief definitions of gluten, a list where it can be found and a detailed list of ingredients found in cosmetics and body care products that contain gluten.

Section 2: Is an itemized list of personal care products and brands. Simply use the Table of Contents to direct you to the type of personal care product you are interested in and go to that page.

 Example: page 44 is Deodorants
- All the brands are in alphabetical order.
- Under each brand name are the products they carry.
- The list will tell you if the product is gluten-free (GF) or not.
- The far right column, labeled, "Company Information" provides you with the response I received directly from the company.
- Page 15 provides a list of key terms used.

Take this handbook with you to the store so that you can be confident that the products you are purchasing are safe. If you have any doubts, please contact the company directly. Companies are always revamping the lines, so please refer to their websites.

---

eZ Gluten-Free Life web information:

Web page	www.ezglutenfreelife.com
Blog	ezglutenfreelife.blogspot.com
Pinterest	http://pinterest.com/ezglutenfreelif/
FaceBook	https://www.facebook.com/EZGlutenFreeLife?ref=hl

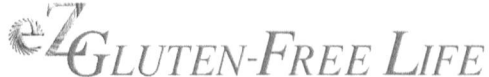

Table of Contents.

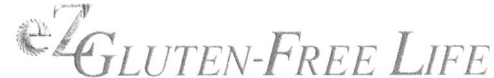
Everyone is talking about gluten these days. You cannot open a magazine or listen to a news report without gluten inching its way into the subject. There is change in the air and for those of us who suffer from a gluten-related disorder, this is a very good thing. Until recently, there has been very little known about gluten-related diseases. Research has been limited to those few doctors willing to fight for what they believe in. But in the last few years things have begun to shift. Testing has improved dramatically and doctors are becoming more aware of the medical issues gluten can cause.

Gluten has many different meanings, depending on who you are. Webster defines gluten as, "gray, sticky, nutritious substances found in wheat flour." My friend is a bread baker and to him, gluten is the substance that adds elasticity to baked goods, it helps the baked goods rise and makes the baked goods chewy. To Celiac or Hashimoto's patient, gluten is the substance that makes them feel sick.

Gluten is the protein associated with autoimmune diseases, Celiac disease, Dermatitis Herpetiformis, Gluten Ataxia, gluten sensitivities and Hashimoto's. The specific gluten that causes these disorders and diseases can be found in **wheat, barley, rye** (sometimes known as WBR) **and possibly oats,** (due to cross contamination) and products made with these ingredients. Dr. Peter Green, author of *Celiac Disease, A Hidden Epidemic*, states that, "Gluten is the term for the storage protein of wheat. Wheat is approximately 10 to 15 percent protein; remainder is starch. Gluten is what remains after the starch granules are washed from the wheat flour." (Green, p. 21)

The term "gluten" has become a generic term for the specific gluten found in wheat, barley and rye which causes damage to the body, if a person is sensitive to it. This book uses the word "gluten" to refer to gluten found in **wheat, barley, rye and possibly oats.** The same is usually true when recipe books, food labels, blogs, etc. use the word gluten. There is more than one type of gluten. Gliadin is a storage protein found in **wheat.** Secalin is the storage protein found in **rye.** Hordein is the storage protein found in **barley.** These specific storage proteins are the gluten proteins that are associated with Celiac and other gluten intolerances.

As research improves the array of disorders, diseases and medical issues believed to be affected by gluten is growing. Several of the well known disorders/diseases are:

Celiac disease (CD), is also known as celiac sprue or gluten-sensitive enteropathy. It is an autoimmune disease which is genetic and therefore inherited disease. It affects people of all ages and is believed that approximately 1 in 141 people have Celiac disease, yet most are undiagnosed. When gluten is eaten the small intestine becomes damaged. The villi are pushed down by the gluten creating an environment that is unable to absorb nutrients. There are over 300 registered symptoms for Celiac. The most common symptoms are diarrhea, bloating, anemia, chronic fatigue, weakness, bone pain, weight loss and muscle cramps. It was once thought that Celiac's only affect the small intestine but it is now known that it can causes a variety of medical issues. (Green p.2-4)

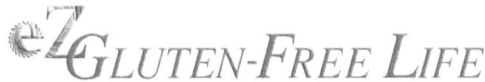
Dermatitis Herpetiformis is the same disease as Celiac but the symptoms manifest themselves under the skin causing "groups of watery, itchy blisters that may resemble pimples or blisters."(gluten.net #29). Dermatitis herpetiformis is usually the primary symptom and the small intestinal symptoms are reduced. (gluten.net # 29)

Autoimmune Disease: Research has begun to prove that many autoimmune diseases are triggered or affected by the consumption of gluten.

Hashimoto's is an autoimmune thyroid disorder. It is believed that when gluten is eaten the body believes it is a foreign substance and sends histamines to attack the gluten. The histamines can mistake the thyroid for gluten and attack it instead. (Kharrazian, p.5-8)

Gluten Ataxia is when gluten toxins affect the brain causing neurological problems such as balance issues, coordination and speech problems. (Boyd. Pg 4)

Non-Celiac Gluten Sensitivity symptoms are similar to Celiac, but unlike Celiac's, the symptoms extend past the digestive system. Symptoms include brain fog, headaches, joint pain, numbness of the arms & legs, muscle cramps, and chronic fatigue.

This is not an exhausted list.

Personal Care Products:
Can gluten in personal care products harm you?

Personal Care Products such as cosmetics and body care products can contain gluten and many of them do. There is some debate about whether or not this is an issue for people with Celiac Disease, Autoimmune Diseases, Dermatitis Herpetiformis, Gluten Ataxia, Hashimoto's and gluten sensitivities. Most doctors suggest that these people avoid gluten, no matter the form it is in.

There are two trains of thought about gluten in products that touch our skin. Some doctors believe that the gluten molecule is too large to cross the skin barrier and therefore will not affect a person with gluten issues. Others doctors believe that what we put on our skin directly affects what is going on inside our bodies.

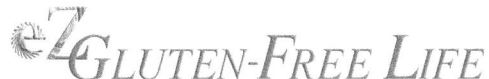

GLUTEN-FREE LIFE

There is another issue, especially for those with gluten intolerant issues that affect the skin such as psoriasis, eczema and Dermatitis Herpetiformis. These skins reactions can occur when someone sensitive to gluten ingests gluten and/or touches gluten. For me and so many other people I have communicated with, the simple act of putting a product that contains gluten on their skin will set off a reaction.

There are cosmetics, such as lipstick and eye makeup, which can easily be absorbed into the body. Shampoos and conditioners containing gluten can run down the face and into the mouth causing gluten reactions. Toothpastes with gluten can have the same reaction as if a person eats the gluten. Products in spray form such as: hair spray, perfume, or body mist can contain gluten. When spraying products containing gluten molecules, gluten is released in the air. These molecules can be breathed in and affect a person sensitive to gluten. It is important to read all ingredient labels before using these products.

Unlike food products, the FDA does not yet have regulations for allergen labeling rules for personal care products. This means they are not required to highlight, or point out if a product contains Wheat, Barley, Rye, and Oats or any of the 8 major allergens. This can lead to gluten exposure and cross contamination. Nor do they have to state if the product has been produced in the same facility as allergens.

It is difficult to find the gluten ingredients in these products because scientific compounds are often used. These ingredients may be found in body care products such as soaps, shampoos, deodorant, cosmetics, nail products, sun screen, toothpastes, and lip gloss, etc. An extensive list of gluten ingredients found in these products is included in this guide. If you have any doubts about the products, it is important that you write or call the companies to confirm the use of gluten in the products and their cross contamination procedures in the production of the products.

Please note that after talking to numerous perfume/cologne companies I realized that most of them do not have any ingredient and allergen information available.

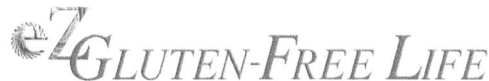

You will rarely find the word gluten written in the ingredients list. Oh, if it where that simple. Wheat, barley and rye (WBR) also have genus names which may be used in the ingredients list. In addition, there are many forms of wheat, some which do not include the word wheat. *Gluten-Free Living 101 Handbook* goes into detail about the diseases, alternative names for gluten, how to read labels and the products that may be harboring gluten. For this handbook, the basic alternative names for wheat, barley and rye have been included.

Alternative Names for Wheat, Barley and Rye

Barley: genus Hordeum

For more information: http://www.gramene.org/species/hordeum/barley_intro.html

Other Names for Barley:

Barley Grass	Pearl Barley
Barley *Hordeum Vulgare*	Malt or Malt Flavoring
Barley Malt or Malt Barley	Caramel Coloring (can be made with malt barley)

Oat: genus Avena (*Celiac patients and people who have been told to avoid cross contamination need to eat gluten- free oats and follow Celiac Spruce protocol unless otherwise instructed by a physician. Please refer to this website for further information.*)

http://www.csaceliacs.info/guide_to_oats.jsp*)*

According to www.livingwithout.com, pure, uncontaminated oats (up to ½ cup dry oats daily) can be tolerated by most celiac patients.

Rye: genus Secale

For more information: http://www.gramene.org/species/secale/rye_intro.html

Triticale (wheat/rye hybrid)

For more information: ftp://ftp.fao.org/docrep/fao/009/y5553e/y5553e01.pdf

Wheat: genus Triticum

Other names for wheat:

Bulgur	Gliadin	Wheat Berry
Couscous	Gluten Peptides	Wheat Germ
Dinkle	Graham	Wheat Germ Oil
Durum	Kamut	Wheat Gluten
Emmer	Seitan	Wheatgrass
Faro	Semolina	Wheat Nut
Fu	Spelt	Wheat Starch

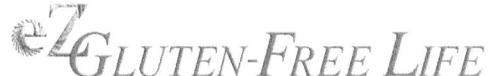

ℯℤGLUTEN-FREE LIFE

It is difficult to find the gluten ingredients in these products because often the scientific name is used for the ingredients. It is important that you write to certain companies to confirm their cross contamination procedures in the production of their products, if you have any doubts.

These are alternative names for ingredients found in body care products that are sources of gluten. These may be found in body care products such as soaps, shampoos, deodorant, cosmetics, sun screen, toothpastes, and lip gloss, etc. This may not be a complete list.

Key words to look for:

Wheat   *Avena Sativa*
Rye   Hydrolyzed...
Barley   *Triticum Vulgare*
Malt
Oat (unless labeled gluten free)

▲ = COSMETIC INGREDIENTS THAT MAY CONTAIN GLUTEN*

▲ Amino Peptide Complex
▲ AMP-Isostearoyl Hydrolyzed Wheat Protein
▲ AMP-Isostearoyl Wheat/Corn/Soy Amino Acids
▲ Aspergillus/Saccharomyces/Barley Ferment Extract Filtrate
▲ Aspergillus/Saccharomyces/Barley Seed Ferment Extract
▲ Aspergillus/Saccharomyces/Barley Seed Ferment Filtrate Extract
▲ Aspergillus/Saccharomyces/Wheat Lees Ferment Filtrate
▲ Aspergillus/Soybean/Wheat Germ/Camellia Sinensis Leaf/Job's Tears Seed/Rice Germ /Sesame Seed Ferment
▲ Aspergillus/Soybean/Wheat Germ/Camellia Sinensis Leaf/Job's Tears Seed/Rice Germ /Sesame Seed Ferment Extract
▲ Avena Sativa (Oat) Bran
▲ Avena Sativa (Oat) Bran Extract
▲ Avena Sativa (Oat) Kernel Extract
▲ Avena Sativa (Oat) Kernel Meal
▲ Avena Sativa (Oat) Kernel Oil
▲ Avena Sativa (Oat) Kernel Protein
▲ Avena Sativa (Oat) Leaf Extract
▲ Avena Sativa (Oat) Meal Extract
▲ Avena Sativa (Oat) Peptide
▲ Avena Sativa (Oat) Protein Extract
▲ Avena Sativa (Oat) Starch
▲ Avena Sativa (Oat) Straw Extract

GLUTEN-FREE LIFE

- ▲ Bacillus/Wheat Bran/Phaseolus Angularis Seed/Prunus Armeniaca Seed/Artemisia Annua Extract/Xanthium Strumarium Fruit Extract/Glycine Soja Seed Ferment Extract
- ▲ Barley (Hordeum Distichim) Extract
- ▲ Barley (Hordeum Distichum) Flour
- ▲ Barley (Hordeum Vulgare) Extract
- ▲ Barley (Hordeum Vulgare) Flour
- ▲ Barley (Hordeum Vulgare) Juice
- ▲ Barley (Hordeum Vulgare) Leaf Juice
- ▲ Barley (Hordeum Vulgare) Powder
- ▲ Barley (Hordeum Vulgare) Root Extract
- ▲ Barley (Hordeum Vulgare) Seed Extract
- ▲ Barley Derived Ingredients (Flour)
- ▲ Barley Extract
- ▲ Barley Juice
- ▲ Barley Leaf Juice
- ▲ Barley Seed Flour
- ▲ Cetearyl Wheat Bran Glycosides
- ▲ Cetearyl Wheat Straw Glycosides
- ▲ Cocodimonium Hydroxypropyl Hydrolyzed Wheat Protein
- ▲ Cocoyl Hydrolyzed Wheat Protein
- ▲ Cycoldextrin
- ▲ Disodium Wheat Germamido MEASulfosuccinate
- ▲ Disodium Wheat Germamido PEG-2 Sulfosuccinate
- ▲ Disodium Wheatgermamphodiacetate
- ▲ Ethyl Wheat Germate
- ▲ Extract of Barley
- ▲ Extract of Barley Root
- ▲ Extract of Barley Seed
- ▲ Hordeum Distichon (Barley) Extract
- ▲ Hordeum Distichon (Barley) Seed Flour
- ▲ Hydrogenated Wheat Germ Oil
- ▲ Hydrogenated Wheat Germ Oil Unsaponifiables
- ▲ Hydrolyzed Barley Protein
- ▲ Hydrolyzed Oat Flour
- ▲ Hydrolyzed Oat Protein
- ▲ Hydrolyzed Oats
- ▲ Hydrolyzed Rye Phytoplacenta Extract
- ▲ Hydrolyzed Wheat Bran
- ▲ Hydrolyzed Wheat Flour

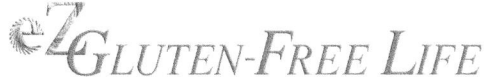

▲ Hydrolyzed Wheat Gluten
▲ Hydrolyzed Wheat Gluten Extract
▲ Hydrolyzed Wheat Protein Hydroxypropyl Polysiloxane
▲ Hydrolyzed Wheat Protein PG-Propyl Methylsilanediol
▲ Hydrolyzed Wheat Protein PG-Propyl Silanetriol
▲ Hydrolyzed Wheat Protein/Cystine Bis- PG-Propyl Silanetriol Copolymer
▲ Hydrolyzed Wheat Protein/Dimethicone PEG-7 Acetate
▲ Hydrolyzed Wheat Protein/Dimethicone PEG-7 Phosphate Copolymer
▲ Hydrolyzed Wheat Protein/PEG-20 Acetate Copolymer
▲ Hydrolyzed Wheat Protein/PVP Crosspolymer
▲ Hydrolyzed Wheat Starch
▲ Hydroxypropyltrimonium Corn/Wheat/Soy Amino Acids Hydroxypropyltrimonium
   Hydrolyzed Wheat Protein
▲ Hydroxypropyltrimonium Hydrolyzed Wheat Protein/Siloxysilicate
▲ Hydroxypropyltrimonium Hydrolyzed Wheat Starch
▲ Kluyveromyces/Lactobacillus/Lactococcus/Leuconostoc/
   Saccharomyces/Hydrolyzed Wheat Protein Ferment Filtrate
▲ Lactobacillus/Oat/Rye/Wheat Seed Extract Ferment
▲ Lactobacillus/Rye Flour Ferment
▲ Lactobacillus/Rye Flour Ferment Filtrate
▲ Laurdimonium Hydroxypropyl Hydrolyzed Wheat Protein
▲ Laurdimonium Hydroxypropyl Hydrolyzed Wheat Protein/Siloxysilicate
▲ Laurdimonium Hydroxypropyl Hydrolyzed Wheat Protein/Siloxysilicate
▲ Laurdimonium Hydroxypropyl Hydrolyzed Wheat Starch
▲ Laurdimonium Hydroxypropyl Wheat Amino Acids
▲ Malt Extract
▲ Maltitol
▲ Maltose
▲ Oat (*Avena Sativa*) Extract
▲ Oat Amino Acids
▲ Oat Beta Glucanoat Extract
▲ Oat Derived Ingredients (Bran, Flour, Oatmeal)
▲ Oat Floursodium Lauroyl
▲ Oat Gum
▲ Olivoyl Hydrolyzed Wheat Protein
▲ Palmitoyl Hydrolyzed Wheat Protein
▲ Pantoea Agglomerans/Wheat Flour Ferment Extract
▲ PG-Hydrolyzed Wheat Protein
▲ Polygonum Fagopyrum (Buckwheat) Leaf Extract
▲ Potassium Cocoyl Hydrolyzed Oat Protein

▲ Potassium Cocoyl Hydrolyzed Wheat Protein
▲ Potassium Lauroyl Wheat Amino Acids
▲ Potassium Olivoyl Hydrolyzed Wheat Protein
▲ Potassium Olivoyl/Lauroyl Wheat Amino Acids
▲ Potassium Palmitoyl Hydrolyzed Oat Protein
▲ Potassium Palmitoyl Hydrolyzed Wheat Protein
▲ Potassium Undecylenoyl Hydrolyzed Wheat Protein
▲ Propyltrimonium Hydrolyzed Wheat Protein
▲ Quaternium-79 Hydrolyzed Wheat Protein
▲ Rye Extract
▲ Rye Flour
▲ Rye Seed Extract
▲ Rye Seed Flour
▲ Saccharomcyes/Barley Seed Ferment Extract
▲ Saccharomyces/Barley Seed Ferment Filtrate
▲ Samino Peptide Complex
▲ Savena Sativa (Oat) Flour
▲ Secale Cereale (Rye Product)
▲ Secale Cereale (Rye) Phyto Placenta Culture Extract Filtrate
▲ Secale Cereale (Rye) Phyto Placenta Culture Extract Filtrate
▲ Secale Cereale (Rye) Seed Extract
▲ Secale Cereale (Rye) Seed Flour
▲ Sodium C8-16 Isoalkylsuccinyl Wheat Sulfonate
▲ Sodium Capryloyl Hydrolyzed Wheat Protein
▲ Sodium Cocoyl Hydrolyzed Wheat Protein
▲ Sodium Cocoyl Hydrolyzed Wheat Protein Glutamate
▲ Sodium Cocoyl Hydrolyzed Wheat Protein Glutamate
▲ Sodium Cocoyl Oat Amino Acids
▲ Sodium Lauroyl Oat Amino Acids
▲ Sodium Lauroyl Wheat Amino Acids
▲ Sodium Palmitoyl Hydrolyzed Wheat Protein
▲ Sodium Palmitoyl Hydrolyzed Wheat Protein
▲ Sodium Stearoyl Hydrolyzed Wheat Protein
▲ Sodium Stearoyl Hydrolyzed Wheat Protein
▲ Sodium Stearoyl Oat Protein
▲ Sodium Wheat Germamphoacetate
▲ Sodium/TEA-Undecylenoyl Hydrolyzed Wheat Protein
▲ Sodium/TEA-Undecylenoyl Hydrolyzed Wheat Protein
▲ Soyamidoethyldimonium/Trimonium Hydroxypropyl Hydrolyzed Wheat Protein
▲ Soydimonium Hydroxypropyl Hydrolyzed Wheat Protein

▲ Soydimonium Hydroxypropyl Hydrolyzed Wheat Protein
▲ Steardimonium Hydroxypropyl Hydrolyzed Wheat Protein
▲ Stearyldimonium Hydroxypropyl Hydrolyzed Wheat Protein
▲ Streptococcus Zooepidemicus/Wheat Peptide Ferment
▲ Tocopherol/Wheat Polypeptides
▲ Trimethylsilyl Hydrolyzed Wheat Protein PG-Propyl Methylsilanediol Crosspolymer
▲ Triticum Aestivum (Wheat) Flour Lipids
▲ Triticum Aestivum (Wheat) Germ Extract
▲ Triticum Aestivum (Wheat) Germ Oil
▲ Triticum Aestivum (Wheat) Leaf Extract
▲ Triticum Aestivum (Wheat) Peptide
▲ Triticum Aestivum (Wheat) Seed Extract
▲ Triticum Turgidum Durum (Wheat) Seed Extract
▲ Triticum Vulgare (Wheat) Bran
▲ Triticum Vulgare (Wheat) Bran Extract
▲ Triticum Vulgare (Wheat) Bran Lipids
▲ Triticum Vulgare (Wheat) Flour Extract
▲ Triticum Vulgare (Wheat) Flour Lipids
▲ Triticum Vulgare (Wheat) Germ
▲ Triticum Vulgare (Wheat) Germ Extract
▲ Triticum Vulgare (Wheat) Germ Oil
▲ Triticum Vulgare (Wheat) Germ Oil Unsaponifiables
▲ Triticum Vulgare (Wheat) Germ Powder
▲ Triticum Vulgare (Wheat) Germ Protein
▲ Triticum Vulgare (Wheat) Gluten
▲ Triticum Vulgare (Wheat) Gluten Extract
▲ Triticum Vulgare (Wheat) Kernel Flour
▲ Triticum Vulgare (Wheat) Protein
▲ Triticum Vulgare (Wheat) Seed Extract
▲ Triticum Vulgare (Wheat) Sprout Extract
▲ Triticum Vulgare (Wheat) Starch
▲ Undecylenoyl Wheat Amino Acids
▲ Vitamin E Derived From Wheat Germ Oil
▲ Wheat Amino Acids
▲ Wheat Derived Ingredients (Bran, Flour)
▲ Wheat Germ Acid
▲ Wheat Germ Extract
▲ Wheat Germ Glycerides
▲ Wheat Germ Oil PEG-40 Butyloctanol Esters
▲ Wheat Germ Oil PEG-8 Esters

▲ Wheat Germ Oil/Palm Oil Aminopropanediol Esters
▲ Wheat Germamide DEA
▲ Wheat Germamidopropalkonium Chloride
▲ Wheat Germamidopropyl Betaine
▲ Wheat Germamidopropyl Dimethylamine
▲ Wheat Germamidopropyl Dimethylamine Lactate
▲ Wheat Germamidopropyl Epoxypropyldimonium Chloride
▲ Wheat Germamidopropylamine Oxide
▲ Wheat Germamidopropyldimonium Hydroxypropyl Hydrolyzed Wheat Protein
▲ Wheat Gluten
▲ Wheat Protein
▲ Wheat Protein Hydrolysate
▲ Wheatgermamidopropyl Dimethylamine Hydrolyzed Collagen
▲ Wheatgermamidopropyl Dimethylamine Hydrolyzed Wheat Protein
▲ Wheatgermamidopropyl Dimethylamine Hydrolyzed Wheat Protein
▲ Wheatgermamidopropyl Ethyldimonium Ethosulfate
▲ Wheat Starch
▲ Yeast Extract
▲ Zea Mays (Corn) Gluten Protein
▲ Zinc Undecylenoyl Hydrolyzed Wheat Protein

References:
1. "The CSA Gluten-Free Product Listing, 14th Edition".
   Celiac Sprue Association. Omaha, NE. 2010. PAGE 15
2. https://ftp.epowercenterdirect.com/LorealContent/gluten%
   20list%20for%20Consumer%20Site%20Redken.pdf
3. Emails from numerous companies.

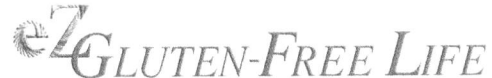

e^ZGluten-Free Life

Key Terms	Definitions
GF	Gluten Free
Variables	
CC	Cross Contamination: Product may have been exposed to gluten during the manufacturing process.
GLUTEN	Definitely contains gluten
GLUTEN/CC	Product contains gluten or has been exposed to cross contamination.
Possible CC	Contains no gluten ingredients but has not been tested for CC.
READ	Read the company information in the far right column.
Undetermined	Line is too extensive. Email or call about specific product.

Disclaimer:

Please remember this reference guide is meant to be used as an informative guide and is in no way meant to replace or conflict with medical advice of physicians. Always check the labels, ingredients and allergen warnings before consuming any food product or using any product that may come in contact with your body. Ingredients and formulas can change at any time. Regulations vary from country to country, so products listed as gluten-free in the U.S. may not be gluten-free in other countries.

Many ingredient labels appear NOT to have gluten in them yet during the company's communication to me, the company either does not list them as gluten-free or they stated that the product has not been tested and/or certified gluten-free. This especially occurs with non- food products. I have listed these products as: "Contains no gluten ingredients but has not been tested for CC." (CC = Cross Contamination)

This handbook includes a large cross section of companies and brands. New companies and products are introduced continually and other products discontinued on a regular basis. This handbook is not an exhaustive list.

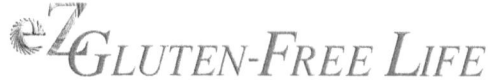

BODY CARE PRODUCTS (GENERAL)	GF	VARIABLES
100% Pure	GF	
365 Premium Body Care	GF	
Afterglow	GF	
Alba Botanica		READ
Arbonne	GF	
Aubrey		Undetermined
Aveeno		Contains Oats
Boots/ Sold at Target	GF	READ
		EXCEPT
		EXCEPT
Botanic Products sold at Target		READ
Organic Body Wash	GF	
Burt's Bees		Undetermined
Clinique		Undetermined
Dakota Free	GF	
Desert Essences Organics	GF	READ
Dove	GF	
Dr. Bronner	GF	
EO	GF	
Giovanni		Undetermined
Gillette Company		READ
Skin Care (All)	GF	
Olay Pro X Products (All)	GF	
Personal Cleansing (All)	GF	
Gillette Body Washes (All)	GF	
Honeybee Gardens	GF	**EXCEPT**
Hugo Naturals	GF	
VERIFIED 2013		

COMPANY INFORMATION

http://www.100percentpure.com/Articles.asp?ID=146

▲ GIG certified Whole Foods Brand

http://www.afterglowcosmetics.com/gluten_free_cosmetics/

www.albabotanica.com

▲ "Our plant-based formulations come from a variety of sources and combinations of derivatives and are not screened for traces of specific allergens. We cannot guarantee that our products are gluten-free."

www.arbonne.com

Line to extensive. Contact Company about specific product.

www.aveeno.com

▲ As per an email response these 2 products in the Boots line contain GLUTEN.

Dual Eye Make Up Remover contents (Triticum Vulgare Protein) wheat

No7 Moisture Drench Lipstick contains wheat germ

▲ As per an email response: These are the only 3 products that are GF in the Botanic Products Line.

http://www.burtsbees.com/u/footernav/need-help/faqs.html#10

Line to extensive. Contact Company about specific product.

▲ Company stated unable to answer question.

https://dakotafree.com/Category.asp?Category_Id=5

(Most of the regular line and all of the Organic line is GF)

http://www.desertessence.com/faqs

http://www.dove.us/Contact-Us/

ALL PRODUCTS GF. www.dbonner.com

GIF certified www.eoproducts.com

Line to extensive. Contact Company about specific product.

▲ Gillette works with many vendors who supply ingredients and can not comment on their other products.

▲ http://www.honeybeegardens.com/

"I'm happy to report that our entire line, with the exception of our hair spray, is gluten-free. AND we are working on the hair spray to make that gluten-free as well."

http://hugonaturals.com/about-our-products

ALWAYS READ INGREDIENTS LABELS!!!

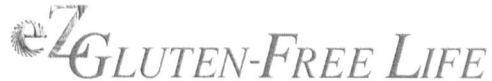

BODY CARE PRODUCTS (GENERAL)	GF	VARIABLES
Jane Cosmetics		Undetermined
Jason		READ
Johnson Baby Hand & Face Wipes	GF	
Johnson and Johnson		Undetermined
Kissmyface		
Moisturizers	GF	
Vitamin A&E Moisturizer	GF	
Honey & Calendula Moisturizer	GF	
Peaches & Crème Moisturizer	GF	
Mill Creek		Contains Oats
Monkey Sea Monkey Doo	GF	
Neutrogena		Undetermined
Nourish	GF	
Nu Skin	GF	
		EXCEPT
VERIFIED 2013		

COMPANY INFORMATION

Line to extensive. Contact Company about specific product.

▲ Read labels some of the products do contain wheat

"Our Plant-based formulations come from a variety of sources and combinations of derivatives and are not screened for traces of specific allergens. We cannot guarantee that our products are gluten-free."

Matison/Matison page 526

▲ While we perform comprehensive testing on the more common ingredients that may provide an allergic reaction such as gluten, nuts etc., unfortunately, it is impossible to test for every ingredient and we cannot guarantee that our products are gluten-free, since the source of an ingredient may change from time to time. Some of the ingredients in the product may have been purchased by us from outside distributors and we cannot say with absolute certainty that cross contamination with this ingredient did not occur at their facilities.

www.kissmyface.com

www.millcreekbotanicals.com

monkeyseamonkeydoo.com (dedicated facility)

Line to extensive. Contact Company about specific product.

www.NourishUSDA.com

www.nuskin.com

▲ All Products GF Except:
AHA Facial Peel (oat kernel extract)
Face Lift Activator, Sensitive skin (wheat)
Face Lift Powder, Sensitive skin (wheat)
Face Lift Powder with Activator, Sensitive skin (wheat)
Tri-Phasic White Essence
Balancing Shampoo (wheat)
Epoch Baby Hibiscus (oat kernel extract)
Moisturizing Shampoo (wheat)
StylinGel (wheat)
Nutriol Shampoo

ALWAYS READ INGREDIENTS LABELS!!!

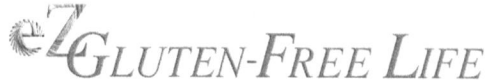

BODY CARE PRODUCTS (GENERAL)	GF	VARIABLES
Oil of Olay		Undetermined
Olivina	GF	
Organique by Himalaya Herbals		READ
Origins		Undetermined
Rainbow Research	GF	
Pangea Organics	GF	
Shiseido	GF	
Zosia Organics	GF	

BODY LOTION	GF	VARIABLES
100% Pure	GF	
365 Premium Body Care	GF	
Afterglow	GF	
Alba Botanica		READ
Arbonne	GF	
Aubrey		Undetermined
Aveeno		Contains Oats
Boots/ Sold at Target	GF	READ
		EXCEPT
		EXCEPT
Burt's Bees		Undetermined
Clean and Clear (Johnson & Johnson)		Undetermined
Clinique		Undetermined
Dakota Free	GF	
Desert Essences Organics	GF	READ

VERIFIED 2013

COMPANY INFORMATION

Line to extensive. Contact Company about specific product.

http://www.olivinanapavalley.com/

▲ All GF products labeled with a green label (Shampoo has wheat)

Line to extensive. Contact Company about specific product.

Some products contain colliodal oats

http://www.pangeaorganics.com

www.sheiseido.com

GIG certified

COMPANY INFORMATION

http://www.100percentpure.com/Articles.asp?ID=146

▲ GIG certified Whole Foods Brand

http://www.afterglowcosmetics.com/gluten_free_cosmetics/

www.albabotanica.com

▲ "Our plant-based formulations come from a variety of sources and combinations of derivatives and are not screened for traces of specific allergens. We cannot guarantee that our products are gluten-free."

www.arbonne.com

Line to extensive. Contact Company about specific product.

www.aveeno.com

▲ As per an email response these 2 products in the Boots line contain GLUTEN.

Dual Eye Make Up Remover contents (Triticum Vulgare Protein) wheat

No7 Moisture Drench Lipstick contains wheat germ

http://www.burtsbees.com/u/footernav/need-help/faqs.html#10

Line to extensive. Contact Company about specific product.

www.cleanandclear.com

▲ Company stated unable to answer question.

https://dakotafree.com/Category.asp?Category_Id=5

(Most of the regular line and all of the Organic line is GF)

http://www.desertessence.com/faqs

ALWAYS READ INGREDIENTS LABELS!!!

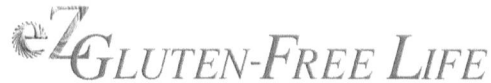
BODY LOTION	GF	VARIABLES
Dove	GF	
Dr. Bronner	GF	
Ecco Bella	GF	
EO	GF	
Eucerin		
Skin Calming Products		Contain Oats
Daily Moisturizing Products		READ
Soothing Products		READ
Intensive Repair		READ
Giovanni		Undetermined
Gillette Company		READ
Skin Care (All)	GF	
Jason		READ
Johnson and Johnson		Undetermined
Kissmyface		**GLUTEN/CC**
Mill Creek		Contains Oats
Monkey Sea Monkey Doo	GF	
Neutrogena		Undetermined
Nourish	GF	
VERIFIED 2013		

COMPANY INFORMATION

http://www.dove.us/Contact-Us/

ALL PRODUCTS GF. www.dbonner.com

http://www.eccobella.com/frequently-asked-questions

GIF certified www.eoproducts.com

"Contains no gluten ingredients but has not been tested for for Cross Contamination. Formulas are changed often. Read Labels."

Line to extensive. Contact Company about specific product.

▲ Gillette works with many vendors who supply ingredients and can not comment on their other products.

http://www.jason-natural.com/body-loving-products

▲ Read labels some of the products do contain wheat

"Our Plant-based formulations come from a variety of sources and combinations of derivatives and are not screened for traces of specific allergens. We cannot guarantee that our products are gluten-free."

▲ While we perform comprehensive testing on the more common ingredients that may provide an allergic reaction such as gluten, nuts etc., unfortunately, it is impossible to test for every ingredient and we cannot guarantee that our products are gluten-free, since the source of an ingredient may change from time to time. Some of the ingredients in the product may have been purchased by us from outside distributors and we cannot say with absolute certainty that cross contamination with this ingredient did not occur at their facilities.

www.kissmyface.com

Kissmyface sent me a detailed list of their GF items and there was NO lotion on the list.

www.millcreekbotanicals.com

monkeyseamonkeydoo.com (dedicated facility)

Line to extensive. Contact Company about specific product.

www.NourishUSDA.com

ALWAYS READ INGREDIENTS LABELS!!!

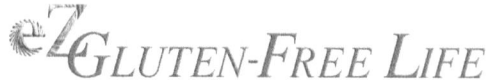

BODY LOTION	GF	VARIABLES
Nu Skin	GF	
		EXCEPT
Oil of Olay		Undetermined
Olivina	GF	
Organique by Himalaya Herbals		READ
Origins		Undetermined
Pangea Organics	GF	
Shiseido	GF	
Zosia Organics	GF	

BODY SOAP (BAR & LIQUID)	GF	VARIABLES
100 % Pure	GF	
365 Premium Body Care	GF	
Arbonne	GF	
Aveeno		Contains Oats
Boots/ Sold at Target		READ
Botanic Products sold at Target		READ
Organic Body Wash	GF	
VERIFIED 2013		

COMPANY INFORMATION

www.nuskin.com
▲ All Products GF Except:
AHA Facial Peel (oat kernel extract)
Face Lift Activator, Sensitive skin (wheat)
Face Lift Powder, Sensitive skin (wheat)
Face Lift Powder with Activator, Sensitive skin (wheat)
Tri-Phasic White Essence
Balancing Shampoo (wheat)
Epoch Baby Hibiscus (oat kernel extract)
Moisturizing Shampoo (wheat)
StylinGel (wheat)
Nutriol Shampoo

Line to extensive. Contact Company about specific product.

http://www.olivinanapavalley.com/
▲ All GF products labeled with a green label (Shampoo has wheat)

Line to extensive. Contact Company about specific product.

http://www.pangeaorganics.com

www.sheiseido.com

GIG certified

COMPANY INFORMATION

http://www.100percentpure.com/Articles.asp?ID=146

GIG certified Whole Foods Brand

www.arbonne.com

www.aveeno.com
▲ As per an email response these 2 products in the Boots line contain GLUTEN.
Dual eye make up remover contents (Triticum Vulgare Protein) wheat
No7 Moisture Drench Lipstick contains wheat germ.

▲ As per an email response: These are the only 3 products that are GF in the Botanic Products Line.

ALWAYS READ INGREDIENTS LABELS!!!

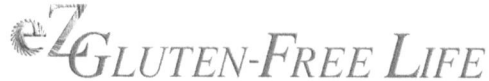

GLUTEN-FREE LIFE

BODY SOAP (BAR & LIQUID)	GF	VARIABLES
Cashmere Bouquet Bar Soap		Undetermined
Dakota Free	GF	
Dr. Bronner	GF	
Desert Essences Organics	GF	
Desert Essences Non organic		Undetermined
Dove	GF	
Dr. Bronner	GF	
Ecover	GF	**EXCEPT**
Gillette Company		READ
Skin Care		
All Olay Pro X Products are Gluten Free		
Personal Cleansing		
All Gillette Body Wash Products are Gluten Free		
Honeybee Gardens	GF	
Hugo Natural	GF	
Irish Spring Bar Soap:		Possible CC
Johnson and Johnson		Undetermined

VERIFIED 2013

COMPANY INFORMATION

"...we do not intentionally add gluten to any of our other products. Though we obtain our ingredients from reliable and trusted suppliers who maintain our high standards for safety, quality, and efficacy, we cannot guarantee that the ingredients used have not come in contact with any gluten."

https://dakotafree.com

www.drbronner.com

Most of our products and all of our Organics line are Gluten Free.

▲ Please refer to packaging to determine if product is gluten free or not.
   http://www.desertessence.com/faqs

http://www.dove.us/Contact-Us/

ALL PRODUCTS GF

▲ http://www.ecover.com/gb/en/allergiesskin.htm
"Are Ecover products suitable for people with gluten intolerance?"

"Wheat is contained in the **Lemon & Aloe Vera washing-up Liquid** and in the **Shower Gel**. Sufferers only normally have a problem if ingested, however some may wish to avoid the wash

▲ Gillette works with many vendors who supply ingredients and can not comment on their other products.

http://www.honeybeegardens.com/

"...we do not intentionally add gluten to any of our other products. Though we obtain our ingredients from reliable and trusted suppliers who maintain our high standards for safety, quality, and efficacy, we cannot guarantee that the ingredients used have not come in contact with any gluten."

▲ While we perform comprehensive testing on the more common ingredients that may provide an allergic reaction such as gluten, nuts etc., unfortunately, it is impossible to test for every ingredient and we cannot guarantee that our products are gluten-free, since the source of an ingredient may change from time to time. Some of the ingredients in the product may have been purchased by us from outside distributors and we cannot say with absolute certainty that cross contamination with this ingredient did not occur at their facilities.

ALWAYS READ INGREDIENTS LABELS!!!

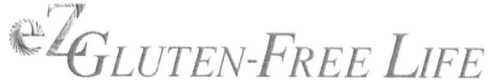

BODY SOAP (BAR & LIQUID)	GF	VARIABLES
Juice Beauty	GF	
Kiss My Face:		
All Olive Oil Bar Soap	GF	
All Liquid Mositure Soaps	GF	
All Self Foaming Soaps	GF	
All Shower Gels	GF	
All Peace Self Foaming Castile Soap	GF	
All Liquid Castile Soap	GF	
Kid's Self Foaming Hand	GF	
Kid's Whale Soap	GF	
Neutrogena		Undetermined
Nourish	GF	
Nu Skin	GF	**EXCEPT**
Olivina	GF	
Organique by Himalaya Herbals		READ
Palmolive Bar Soaps All Variants		Possible CC
Purell	GF	
Rainbow Research	GF	
Softsoap/Liquid		Possible CC.
VERIFIED 2013		

COMPANY INFORMATION

Company sent me a list of all GF items.

Line to extensive. Contact Company about specific product.
www.NourishUSDA.com

▲ www.nuskin.com

All Products GF Except:

AHA Facial Peel (oat kernel extract)

Balancing Shampoo (wheat)

Epoch Baby Hibiscus (oat kernel extract)

Face Lift Activator, Sensitive skin (wheat)

Face Lift Powder, Sensitive skin (wheat)

Face Lift Powder with Activator, Sensitive skin (wheat)

Moisturizing Shampoo (wheat)

StylinGel (wheat)

http://www.olivinanapavalley.com/

▲ All GF products labeled with a green label (Shampoo has wheat)

"...we do not intentionally add gluten to any of our other products. Though we obtain our ingredients from reliable and trusted suppliers who maintain our high standards for safety, quality, and efficacy, we cannot guarantee that the ingredients used have not come in contact with any gluten."

As per an email response

"...we do not intentionally add gluten to any of our other products. Though we obtain our ingredients from reliable and trusted suppliers who maintain our high standards for safety, quality, and efficacy, we cannot guarantee that the ingredients used have not come in contact with any gluten."

ALWAYS READ INGREDIENTS LABELS!!!

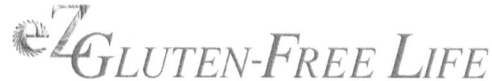

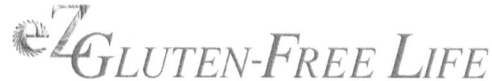*ez* **GLUTEN-FREE LIFE**

BODY SOAP (BAR & LIQUID)	GF	VARIABLES
Softsoap/body washes		Possible CC
Tom's of Maine	GF	**EXCEPT**

COSMETICS	GF	VARIABLES
100% Pure	GF	
Afterglow	GF	
Arbonne	GF	
Aubrey		Undetermined
Aveeno		Contains Oats
Bare Escentuals By Bare Minerals		
		READ
bareMinerals:	GF	
All-Over Face Colors - all shades	GF	
bareEyes Eye Makeup Remover	GF	
Blush - All shades	GF	
Blush (SPF 20) - all shades	GF	
Brushless Mascara	GF	
Body Minerals - all shades	GF	
Eyecolor - all shades	GF	
Extreme Glimmers - all shades	GF	
VERIFIED 2013		

COMPANY INFORMATION

"...we do not intentionally add gluten to any of our other products. Though we obtain our ingredients from reliable and trusted suppliers who maintain our high standards for safety, quality, and efficacy, we cannot guarantee that the ingredients used have not come in contact with any gluten."

▲ All products GF except: (Liquid soap and liquid body soap have gluten) and (New antiperspirant line has gluten)
Natural Moisturizing Body Wash contains wheat protein.

COMPANY INFORMATION

http://www.100percentpure.com/Articles.asp?ID=146

GF & Dedicated facility

www.arbonne.com

Line to extensive. Contact Company about specific product.

www.aveeno.com

http://www.bareescentuals.com/on/demandware.store/5

▲ Which **Bare Escentuals** products are free of Wheat, Oat, Rye and/or Barley derived ingredients? While the list below shows the Wheat, Oat, Rye and Barely free products please keep in mind that these products may be made in an environment that handles Wheat, Oat, Rye and Barley derivatives.

ALWAYS READ INGREDIENTS LABELS!!!

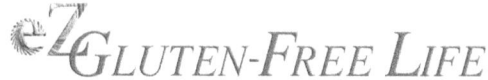

COSMETICS	GF	VARIABLES
bareMinerals continued:	GF	
Faux Tan	GF	
Faux Tan Body Moisturizer	GF	
First Base Lip Balm	GF	
Flawless Definition Mascara - all shades	GF	
Foundation (SPF 15 Original) - all shades	GF	
Foundation (SPF 15 Matte) - all shades	GF	
Gossamers - all shades	GF	
High Shine Eyecolors - all shades	GF	
Hydrating Blush - all shades	GF	
Bare Escentuals BY Bare Minerals		
Liner Shadow - all shades	GF	
Lip Rev-er Upper	GF	
Makeup Remover Wipes	GF	
Mineral Veil - all shades	GF	
Mineral Veil (SPF 25) - all shades	GF	
MultiTasking Minerals - all shades	GF	
On the Spot Swabs	GF	
Prime Time Eyelid Primer	GF	
Prime Time Foundation Primer	GF	
Prime Time Oil Control Foundation Primer	GF	
Quick Change Brush Cleaner	GF	
Radiance Rocks - all shades	GF	
Soft Focus Colors - all shades	GF	
SPF 15 Lipgloss - Fiji	GF	
SPF 30 Natural Sunscreen - all shades	GF	
Weather Everything Liner Sealer	GF	
Well Cared For Brush Shampoo	GF	
BUXOM:		
Buxom Insider Liner - all shades	GF	
Buxom Lash Mascara	GF	
Buxom Lashliner - all shades	GF	
Buxom Lip Polish - all shades	GF	

VERIFIED 2013

COMPANY INFORMATION

http://www.bareescentuals.com/on/demandware.store/5

ALWAYS READ INGREDIENTS LABELS!!!

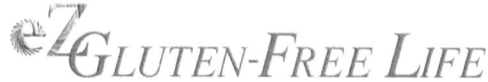

eZ GLUTEN-FREE LIFE

COSMETICS	GF	VARIABLES
Boots/ Sold at Target	GF	READ
		EXCEPT
		EXCEPT
Botanic Products sold at Target		READ
Organic Body Wash	GF	
Organic Rosehip Facial	GF	
Organic Rose Toner	GF	
Clinique		**GLUTEN/ CC**
Cover Girl		**GLUTEN/ CC**
Dakota Free	GF	
Dr. Hauschka (make up only)	GF	
Ecco Bella	GF	
Estee Lauder		**GLUTEN/CC**
Glō·Mineral	GF	
		EXCEPT
Gluten Free Beauty	GF	
Jane Cosmetics		Undetermined
Juice Beauty	GF	
Kiss (Fake eyelashes & adhesive)	GF	
Lancome		Undetermined
La Fresh Wipes	GF	
Larenim	GF	
VERIFIED 2013		

COMPANY INFORMATION

▲ As per an email response these 2 products in the Boots line contain GLUTEN.
Dual Eye Make Up Remover contents (Triticum Vulgare Protein) wheat
No7 Moisture Drench Lipstick contains wheat germ.
▲ As per an email response: These are the only 3 products that are GF in the Botanic
Products Line.

---

www.clinique.com
Line to extensive. Contact Company about specific product.

▲ Owned by Maybelline

https://dakotafree.com/Category.asp?Category_Id=5

http://drhauschka.com/customer-service/faqs.aspx?cid=3#
Make Up is GF but there is gluten in some of the other products.

http://www.eccobella.com/frequently-asked-questions

▲ Smashbox and Estee Lauder are made in the same facility.
Due to the extensive line there are "vast number of raw materials used from different
suppliers etc." Therefore they can not say if there is gluten in the products or whether
go not the products have been exposed to gluten.

http://www.gloprofessional.com/
Face Primer
Lip Filler Pencil
Moisturizing Body Wash
Smoothing Salt Scrub

www.glutenfreebeauty.com
Line to extensive. Contact Company about specific product.

www.janecosmetics.com

http://www.juicebeauty.com/about-organics/faqs#

www.kissusa.com   email response 4/2012

www.lancome.com

▲ Have all natural ingredients and gluten free.
They are great for traveling or someone on the go.
Products include:
Waterproof Make-up Remover
Oil-free Face Cleanser

ALL PRODUCTS GF   http://www.larenim.com/why-larenim

ALWAYS READ INGREDIENTS LABELS!!!

COSMETICS	GF	VARIABLES
M.A.C		READ
Maybelline		**GLUTEN/ CC**
Mineral Fusion	GF	
NARS	GF	
NuSkin	GF	READ **EXCEPT**
Organique by Himalaya Herbals	GF	
		EXCEPT
Origins		Undetermined
Revlon		Undetermined
Sephora		See Website
Shiseido	GF	
Smashbox		READ
Sophtyo	GF	
Wet N Wild	GF	
		EXCEPT
VERIFIED 2013		

COMPANY INFORMATION

▲ "As you may know, our product line is quite extensive. Therefore, in order to respond to your inquiry regarding Gluten, we need to know the exact name and shade of the product(s) which you use or would be interested in using. We will then consult our laboratories and share our findings with you."

https://ftp.epowercenterdirect.com/LorealContent/

www.mineralfusion.com

www.narscosmetics.com

▲ www.nuskin.com

All products are GF except below list:

AHA Facial Peel (oat kernel extract)	Balancing Shampoo (wheat)
Face Lift Activator, Sensitive skin (wheat)	Epoch Baby Hibiscus (oat kernel extract)
Face Lift Powder, Sensitive skin (wheat)	Moisturizing Shampoo (wheat)
Face Lift Powder with Activator,	StylinGel (wheat)
Sensitive skin (wheat)	Nutriol Shampoo
Tri-Phasic White Essence	

▲ All GF products labeled with a green label (Shampoo has wheat) EXCEPT Shampoo which has wheat.

Line to extensive. Contact Company about specific product.

Line to extensive. Contact Company about specific product.

Go to www. sephora.com & put gluten free products in search box - all GF products appear GF at Sephora: Jonathan Products, Alterna, Lavanila, Hourglass & Pacifica Island

www.shiseido.com

▲ Smashbox and Estee Lauder are made in the same facility.
Due the extensive line there are "vast number of raw materials used from different suppliers etc." Therefore they can not say if there is gluten in the products or whether go not the products have been exposed to gluten.

Gluten-free, vegan and organic http://www.sophyto.co.uk/

▲ http://wnwbeauty.com/

Are wet n wild products gluten-free?

Most wet n wild products are gluten-free except for the following:

821A-827A Natural Blend Pressed Powder

745-749 Natural Blend Mineral Foundation and Mineral Veil

C641A MegaProtein Mascara

All other products are gluten-free.

ALWAYS READ INGREDIENTS LABELS!!!

eZ GLUTEN-FREE LIFE

DENTAL (TOOTHPASTE, MOUTH WASH & ORAL CARE PRODUCTS)		GF	VARIABLES
Act by Chattem	Mouth Wash	GF	
Aquafresh	Toothpaste	GF	
Biotene	All Products	GF	
Cepacol		GF	
Colgate	ALL Toothpastes	GF	
	ALL Other Dental Product		Possible CC
Crest	Toothpaste	GF	
	Crest White Strips	GF	
	Crest Night Effects	GF	
	Crest Pro-Health Rinse		Possible CC
	Crest Whitening Rinse		Possible CC
Desert Essence	Natural Tea tree Oil Toothpaste	GF	
Organics	Tea Tree Oil Mouthwash	GF	
Dr. Connor	Whiting	GF	
	Floss	GF	
	Toothpaste	GF	
	Tooth Brush	GF	
	Accessories	GF	
Efferdent	Denture Cleaner	GF	
Effergrip	Denture Adhesive Cleaner	GF	
Glide	Floss	GF	
Glaxo Smith Kline	Sensodyne ProNamel	GF	
	Pronamel Range of Product		**GLUTEN**
Himalaya Herbal Healthcare			
	Neem & Pomegranate Toothpaste,	GF	
Jason	All Toothpastes with "NO Gluten" on box	GF	
Kiss My Face	Sensitive Toothpaste	GF	
	Triple Action Toothpaste	GF	
	Mouthwash	GF	
	Anticavity Toothpaste	GF	
	Toothpaste Whitening Aloe Vera Gel	GF	
	Tartar Control Toothpaste	GF	
VERIFIED 2013			

COMPANY INFORMATION

Contains no gluten but has not been tested
http://www.aquafresh.com/FAQ.aspx

All Colgate Toothpaste is certified gluten-free/
http://www.colgate.com/app/Colgate/US/Corp/ContactUs/
"...we do not intentionally add gluten to any of our other products. Though we obtain our ingredients from reliable and trusted suppliers who maintain our high standards for safety, quality, and efficacy, we cannot guarantee that the ingredients used have not come in contact with any gluten."

https://www.desertessence.com/faqs
https://www.desertessence.com/faqs

1-877-712-9992

ALWAYS READ INGREDIENTS LABELS!!!

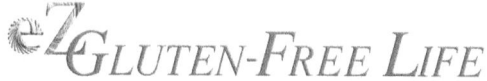

DENTAL (TOOTHPASTE, MOUTH WASH & ORAL CARE PRODUCTS)	GF	VARIABLES
Listerine Agent Cool Blue Tinting Rose	GF	
Antiseptic Mouthwash - all varieties	GF	
Pocket Paks Oral Care Strips- all varieties	GF	
Smart Rinse	GF	
Total Care Anticavity Mouthwash - all varieties	GF	
Whitening (Pen, Pre-Brush Treatment Rinse, Vibrant White Rinse)	GF	
ZERO Mouthwash	GF	
Oral B Oral B Floss	GF	
Oral B Toothpaste	GF	
Orabase Paste by Colgate		Possible CC
Peelu Toothpaste	GF	
Gum	GF	
Peroxyl Rinse by Colgate		Possible CC
Phos-Fhur Rinse By Colgate		Possible CC
Prevident Gel by Colgate Flouride Gel		Possible CC
Rembrandt Deeply White Plus Peroxide	GF	
Premium White Mint	GF	
Plus Peroxide Winter Mint		**GLUTEN**
Scope All Mouthwash	GF	
Tom's Of Maine All Dental Products	GF	
VERIFIED 2013		

COMPANY INFORMATION

http://pggillette.custhelp.com/app/answers/detail/a_id/8848/p/349/
session/L3NpZC9XbnpROWJkbA%3D%3D

"...we do not intentionally add gluten to any of our other products. Though we obtain our ingredients from reliable and trusted suppliers who maintain our high standards for safety, quality, and efficacy, we cannot guarantee that the ingredients used have not come in contact with any gluten."

"...we do not intentionally add gluten to any of our other products. Though we obtain our ingredients from reliable and trusted suppliers who maintain our high standards for safety, quality, and efficacy, we cannot guarantee that the ingredients used have not come in contact with any gluten."

"...we do not intentionally add gluten to any of our other products. Though we obtain our ingredients from reliable and trusted suppliers who maintain our high standards for safety, quality, and efficacy, we cannot guarantee that the ingredients used have not come in contact with any gluten."

"...we do not intentionally add gluten to any of our other products. Though we obtain our ingredients from reliable and trusted suppliers who maintain our high standards for safety, quality, and efficacy, we cannot guarantee that the ingredients used have not come in contact with any gluten."

http://www.tomsofmaine.com/research/not-in-our-products

ALWAYS READ INGREDIENTS LABELS!!!

e^zGLUTEN-FREE LIFE

DENTAL (TOOTHPASTE, MOUTH WASH & ORAL CARE PRODUCTS)	GF	VARIABLES
Ultra Brite by Colgate		
Toothpaste: all variants		Possible CC
Xlear and Spry All Dental Products	GF	
DENTURE PRODUCTS		
CUSHION GRIP® Thermoplastic Denture Adhesive		
Efferdent® Products		
Effergrip® Denture Adhesive	GF	
Efferdent® Denture Cleanser	GF	
Power Clean Crystals™ (Cleanser)	GF	
Sea-Bond Denture Adhesives	GF	
Snug® Dental Cushions	GF	
Polident® Products		
PoliGrip® (Denture Adhesives)	GF	
PoliDent® (Denture Cleaning)	GF	
DENTIST OFFICES (ORAL HYGIENE PRODUCTS)		
Premier Dental All Dental Materials	GF	
DMG America All Dental Materials	GF	
Crosstex's Prophy Paste	GF	
Dentsply Caulk All Dental Materials	GF	
Enamel Pro Fluoride (Topical Gel, Bubblegum,	GF	
Cherry, Orange, & Strawberry)	GF	
Fluoride Varnish		
(Strawberries N Cream, Bubblegum)		
Prophy Paste (All Flavors)	GF	
Glitter Prophy Paste (All Flavors)	GF	
Kolorz Prophy Paste (All Flavors)	GF	
Nupro Fluoride	GF	
Prophy Paste	GF	
Sparkle Prophy Paste (All Flavors)	GF	
SparkleFree Prophy Paste (All Flavors)	GF	
Zap Fluoride Gel	GF	
Ziroxide Prophy Paste	GF	
VERIFIED 2013		

COMPANY INFORMATION

"...we do not intentionally add gluten to any of our other products. Though we obtain our ingredients from reliable and trusted suppliers who maintain our high standards for safety, quality, and efficacy, we cannot guarantee that the ingredients used have not come in contact with any gluten."

Merek Co. 1-800-317-2165
1-877-925-5374

1-800-431-2610
1-877-636-2677

1-866-844-2796

ALWAYS READ INGREDIENTS LABELS!!!

DEODORANT		GF	VARIABLES
365 Premium Body Care			
	ALL	GF	
Andrea Rose	Crystal Stick deodorant	GF	
Aubrey			Undetermined
Axe Effect Deodorant			Undetermined
Burt's Bees	Herbal deodorant	GF	
Colgate	Crystal Clean Stick deodorant	GF	
Crystal	ALL	GF	
Dakota Free	ALL	GF	
Degree	Women's Antiperspirant	GF	
	Women's Deodorant	GF	
	Ultra Clear	GF	
	Pure Petal	GF	
Desert Essences Organics			
	ALL	GF	
Dove	Deodorant	GF	
Dove Men	Antiperspirant		Possible CC
Dove Men	Deodorant		Possible CC
EO	Deodorant	GF	
Gluten-Free Savonnerie			
	Pit stop	GF	
Honeybee Gardens			
	Deodorant Powder	GF	
Irish Spring®			Possible CC
Kiss My Face	Liquid Rock-ALL	GF	
Lady Speed Stick Deodorant & Antiperspirant			Undetermined
Lavera	Deodorant Roll-on	GF	
	Deodorant	GF	
	Men's Deodorant	GF	

VERIFIED 2013

COMPANY INFORMATION

GIG certified Whole Foods Brand

http://www.andrearose.com/about.html
Line to extensive. Contact Company about specific product.
http://www.theaxeeffect.com/faq.html   Axe states that if states that if there is gluten in the product it will be in the ingredient list.
http://www.burtsbees.com/u/footernav/need-help/faqs.html#10
www.colgate .com
www.crystal.com
www.dakotafree.com

▲ (Some of the regular line and all of the Organic line is GF)
http://www.desertessence.com/faqs
www.dove.com
Contains no gluten ingredients but has not been tested for CC.
Contains no gluten ingredients but has not been tested for CC.
www.eoproducts.com

gfsoaps.com

http//www.honeybeegardens.com
Contains no gluten ingredients but has not been tested for CC.
http://www.kissmyface.com/content/landing_soaps
"...we do not intentionally add gluten to any of our other products. Though we obtain our ingredients from reliable and trusted suppliers who maintain our high standards for safety, quality, and efficacy, we cannot guarantee that the ingredients used have not come in contact with any gluten."
www.lavera.com

ALWAYS READ INGREDIENTS LABELS!!!

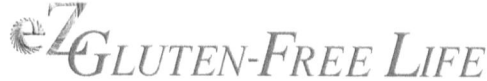

DEODORANT	GF	VARIABLES
Mennen Speed Stick		
Deodorant & Antiperspirant		Undetermined
Nu Skin Deodorant & Antiperspirant	GF	
Nourish Deodorant	GF	
Old Spice All Deodorant	GF	
Secret ALL Products		Undetermined
Speed Stick® Regular	GF	Possible CC
Speed Stick® 24/7®	GF	Possible CC
Speed Stick® Musk	GF	Possible CC
Speed Stick® Ocean Surf®		
Clear	GF	Possible CC
Speed Stick® Power®	GF	Possible CC
Speed Stick® StainGuard®	GF	Possible CC
Tom's of Maine Calendula Deodorant	GF	
Crystal Confidence Roll On	GF	**EXCEPT**
Natural Stick	GF	

FACE CARE PRODUCTS	GF	VARIABLES
100%Pure	GF	
365 Premium Body Care	GF	
Afterglow	GF	
Alba Botanica		READ
Arbonne	GF	
Aubrey		Undetermined
Aveeno		Contains Oats

VERIFIED 2013		

COMPANY INFORMATION

"...we do not intentionally add gluten to any of our other products. Though we obtain our ingredients from reliable and trusted suppliers who maintain our high standards for safety, quality, and efficacy, we cannot guarantee that the ingredients used have not come in contact with any gluten."

https://www.nuskin.com/content/nuskin/en_US/products.html

http//www.nourishusda.com

www.oldspice.com

▲ Secret is owned by PG which is so extensive that they are unable to verify if their products have been exposed to gluten.

Contains no gluten ingredients but has not been tested for CC.

Contains no gluten ingredients but has not been tested for CC.

Contains no gluten ingredients but has not been tested for CC.

Contains no gluten ingredients but has not been tested for CC.

Contains no gluten ingredients but has not been tested for CC.

Contains no gluten ingredients but has not been tested for CC.

www.tomsofmaine.com

▲ All Tom's Antiperspirant Has Gluten

COMPANY INFORMATION

http://www.100percentpure.com/Articles.asp?ID=146

GIG certified   Whole Foods Brand

http://www.afterglowcosmetics.com/gluten_free_cosmetics/

www.albabotanica.com

"Our plant-based formulations come froma variety of sources and combinations of allergens. We cannot guarantee that our products are gluten-free."

www.arbonne.com

Line to extensive. Contact Company about specific product.

www.aveeno.com

ALWAYS READ INGREDIENTS LABELS!!!

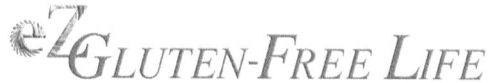

FACE CARE PRODUCTS	GF	VARIABLES
Boots/Sold at Target	GF	READ **EXCEPT** **EXCEPT**
Botanic Products sold at Target		READ
Organic Body Wash	GF	
Organic Rosehip Facial	GF	
Organic Rose Toner	GF	
Burt's Bees		Undetermined
Clean and Clear (Johnson and Johnson)		Undetermined
Clinique		Undetermined
Desert Essences Organics	GF	READ
Dove	GF	
Ecco Bella	GF	
Estee Lauder		Undetermined
Eucerin Face Product Line		READ
Gillette Company		READ
Skin Care (All)	GF	
Olay Pro X Products (All)	GF	
Personal Cleansing (All)	GF	
Gillette Body Washes (All)	GF	
Gluten Free Beauty	GF	
Honeybee Gardens	GF	**EXCEPT**
Jason		READ
VERIFIED 2013		

COMPANY INFORMATION

▲ As per an email response these 2 products in the Boots line contain GLUTEN.
Dual eye make- up remover contents (TriticumVulgare Protein) wheat
No7 Moisture Drench Lipstick contains wheat germ

▲ As per an email response: These are the only 3 products that are GF in the Botanic Products Line.

http://www.burtsbees.com/u/footernav/need-help/faqs.html#10
Line to extensive. Contact Company about specific product.

www.cleanandclear.com

Company stated unable to answer question.

(Most of the regular line and all of the Organic line is GF)
http://www.desertessence.com/faqs

http://www.dove.us/Contact-Us/

http://www.eccobella.com/frequently-asked-questions

Smashbox and Estee Lauder are made in the same facility.
Due to the extensive line there are "vast number of raw materials used from different suppliers etc." Therefore they cannot say if there is gluten in the products or if the products have been exposed to gluten.

Contains no gluten but has not been tested for cross contamination.

Below is a partial list of Gillette's GF products. They work with many vendors who supply ingredients and cannot comment on other pro products

Hair Care
Head & Shoulders (US Shampoos, 2 in1's and Conditioners)
All USA/CA Head & Shoulders products are Gluten Free

www.glutenfreebeauty.com

http://www.honeybeegardens.com/
"I'm happy to report that our entire line, with the exception of our hair spray, is gluten-free. AND we are working on the hair spray to make that gluten-free as well."

http://www.jason-natural.com/body-loving-products
Read labels some of the products do contain wheat

"Our Plant-based formulations come from a variety of sources and combinations of derivatives and are not screened for traces of specific allergens. We cannot guarantee that our products are gluten-free."

ALWAYS READ INGREDIENTS LABELS!!!

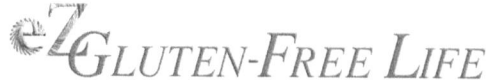

FACE CARE PRODUCTS	GF	VARIABLES
Johnson Baby Hand and Face Wipes	GF	
Johnson and Johnson		Undetermined
Juice Beauty	GF	
Kissmyface:		
Potent & Pure Face Care		
Break Out Botanical Acne Gel	GF	
Brightening Day Crème	GF	
Cell Mate Facial Cream/Sunscreen	GF	
Balancing Act Toner	GF	
Eyewitness Eye Repair Cream	GF	
Pore Shrink Cleansing Mask	GF	
Start Up Exfoliating Face Wash	GF	
Shea Soy Facial Cleansing Bar	GF	
C the Change Ester C Serum	GF	
Clean for a Day Creamy Face Cleanser	GF	
Under Age Ultra Hydrating Moisturizer	GF	
All Tinted Moisturizers	GF	
Lancome		Undetermined
MAC		Undetermined
Mill Creek Botanicals		Contains Oats
NARS	GF	
Neutrogena		Undetermined
Nourish	GF	

VERIFIED 2013

COMPANY INFORMATION

Matison/Matison page 526

While we perform comprehensive testing on the more common ingredients that may provide an allergic reaction such as gluten, nuts etc., unfortunately, it is impossible to test for every ingredient and we cannot guarantee that our products are gluten-free, since the source of an ingredient may change from time to time. Some of the ingredients in the product may have been purchased by us from outside distributors and we cannot say with absolute certainty that cross contamination with this ingredient did not occur at their facilities.

www.juicebeauty.com

www.kissmyface.com

www.lancome.com

Line to extensive. Contact Company about specific product.

Line to extensive. Contact Company about specific product.

www.millcreekbotanicals.com

All Products GF www.narscosmetics.com

Line to extensive. Contact Company about specific product.

www.NourishUSDA.com

ALWAYS READ INGREDIENTS LABELS!!!

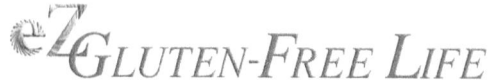

GLUTEN-FREE LIFE

FACE CARE PRODUCTS	GF	VARIABLES
Nu Skin	GF	
		EXCEPT
Oil of Olay		Undetermined
Organique by Himalaya Herbals		READ
Origins		**EXCEPT**
		Undetermined
Pangea Organics	GF	
Shiseido	GF	
Zosia Organics	GF	

HAIR PRODUCTS	GF	VARIABLES
100% Pure	GF	
365 Premium Body Care	GF	
Alterna (Bamboo Line)	GF	**EXCEPT**
Arbonne	GF	
Aubrey		Undetermined
Aveeno		Contains Oats
Bedhead by TIGI (Over 50 ProductsGF. Not all Products GF)		READ
Catwalk by TIGI		**GLUTEN**
VERIFIED 2013		

52

COMPANY INFORMATION

www.nuskin.com
All Products GF Except:
AHA Facial Peel (oat kernel extract)
Face Lift Activator, Sensitive skin (wheat)
Face Lift Powder, Sensitive skin (wheat)
Face Lift Powder with Activator, Sensitive skin (wheat)
Tri-Phasic White Essence
Balancing Shampoo (wheat)
Epoch Baby Hibiscus (oat kernel extract)
Moisturizing Shampoo (wheat)
StylinGel (wheat)
Nutriol Shampoo

Line to extensive. Contact Company about specific product.

http://www.organiquebyhimalaya.com/
All GF products labeled with a green label (Shampoo has wheat)
Line to extensive. Contact Company about specific product.

http://www.pangeaorganics.com

www.sheiseido.com

GIG certified

COMPANY INFORMATION

http://www.100percentpure.com/Articles.asp?ID=146
GIG certified Whole Foods Brand

www.alterna.com. Kenoi oil has wheat.

www.arbonne.com
Line to extensive. Contact Company about specific product.

www.aveeno.com
TIGI sent an email listing the gluten-free products their brands have. The only line is BedHead. Email stated that though some products are GF they cannot guarantee cross contaminated. Please call 800-259-8596 for an extensive list of BedHead GF products.
TIGI states that their only gluten-free line is BedHead.

ALWAYS READ INGREDIENTS LABELS!!!

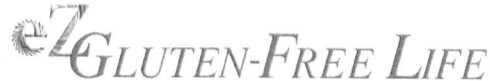

eZ GLUTEN-FREE LIFE

HAIR PRODUCTS	GF	VARIABLES
Clairol		**GLUTEN/CC**
Clinique		Undetermined
Desert Essences Organics	GF	READ
Desert Essences Non Organic		Undetermined
Dove	GF	
		EXCEPT
Dr. Bronner	GF	
Ecologique	GF	
EO	GF	
Garnier		Undetermined
Giovanni		Undetermined
Gillette Company		
Head & Shoulders	GF	
Honeybee Gardens	GF	
		EXCEPT
Hugo Natural	GF	
Jason		READ
Johnson and Johnson		Undetermined
Lancome		Undetermined
L'Oreal		Undetermined
L'Oreal Professional		Undetermined
Matrix		Undetermined
VERIFIED 2013		

COMPANY INFORMATION

www.clariol.com

www.clinique.com

▲ Some of the regular line and all of the Organic line is GF.

http://www.desertessence.com/faqs

http://www.dove.us/Contact-Us/

▲ Daily Treatment

ALL PRODUCTS GF

GIG certified http://formulacorp.com/personal-care/

GIG certified www.eoproducts.com

http://www.garnierusa.com/_en/_us/services/advisor.aspx?isanswerquestion=true

http://www.giovannicosmetics.com/faq.php

▲ Below is a partial list of Gillette's GF products. They work with many vendors who supply ingredients and can not comment on other products.

▲ Head & Shoulders (US Shampoos, 2in1's and Conditioners)
All USA/CA Head & Shoulders products are Gluten Free .

http://www.honeybeegardens.com/

▲ Hairspray has gluten! All other products GF.

The products may have oats that are GF.

▲ Read labels some of the products do contain wheat
"Our Plant-based formulations come from a variety of sources and combinations of derivatives and are not screened for traces of specific allergens. We cannot guarantee that our products are gluten-free."

▲ While we perform comprehensive testing on the more common ingredients that may provide an allergic reaction such as gluten, nuts etc., unfortunately, it is impossible to test for every ingredient and we cannot guarantee that our products are gluten-free, since the source of an ingredient may change from time to time. Some of the ingredients in the product may have been purchased by us from outside distributors and we cannot say with absolute certainty that cross contamination with this ingredient did not occur at their facilities.

Line to extensive. Contact Company about specific product.

Line to extensive. Contact Company about specific product.

▲ http://www.lorealtechnique.com/contact.aspx
"We do not have prepared gluten information for our entire product line."
They do use many gluten products in production.

Line to extensive. Contact Company about specific product.

ALWAYS READ INGREDIENTS LABELS!!!

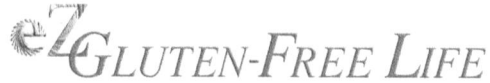

HAIR PRODUCTS	GF	VARIABLES
Method	GF	
Mill Creek		Contains Oats
Morroco Method	GF	
Neutrogena	GF	
Nu Skin	GF	READ **EXCEPT**
Organix		**EXCEPT**
Original Sprout	GF	
PHYTO		**GLUTEN**
Pureology Products		**GLUTEN**
Rainbow Research	GF	
Rene Furterer		Undetermined
Sophyto	GF	
Sauve		**GLUTEN/CC**
S factor by TIGI		**GLUTEN**
TIGI Products		**GLUTEN**
Unite		**GLUTEN/CC**
Weleda		**GLUTEN/CC**
Wen By Chaz Dean		**GLUTEN**

VERIFIED 2013

COMPANY INFORMATION

▲ http://methodhome.com/support/faqs/
"Thanks so much for taking the time to write to us and for your interest in method. Actually, all of our products are gluten free and safe for those with Celiac's disease. We don't use wheat or gluten in any of our ingredients."

www.millcreekbotanicals.com

https://morroccomethod.com/
Line to extensive. Contact Company about specific product.

www.nuskin.com

▲ Balancing Shampoo (wheat)   Face Lift Activator, Sensitive skin (wheat)
   Epoch Baby Hibiscus (oat kernel extract) Face Lift Powder, Sensitive skin (wheat)
   Moisturizing Shampoo (wheat)   Face Lift Powder with Activator,
   StylinGel (wheat)   Sensitive skin (wheat)
   Nutriol Shampoo (wheat)   Tri-Phasic White Essence
   AHA Facial Peel (oat kernel extract)

Biotin and Collagen Line and omit all products are GF.

www.originalsprout.com
100% Vegan, Organic and GF
The majority of the products contain gluten as per email responses.

Read labels as per email

Some products contain colloidal oats

http://www.folica.com/send-contact-us

Certified GF www.sophyto.com

TIGI states that their only gluten-free line is BedHead.
TIGI sent an email listing the gluten-free products their brands have. The only line is BedHead. Email stated that though some products are GF they cannot guarantee cross contaminated. Please call 800-259-8596 for an extensive list of BedHead GF products.

Via email I communicated with the company who claimed their products is gluten free yet I found WHEAT PROTEIN in several of their products.

usa.weleda.com

Contains wheat protein
http://www.wenhaircare.com/whyitsunique.php?mboxSession=1334423515839-7971

ALWAYS READ INGREDIENTS LABELS!!!

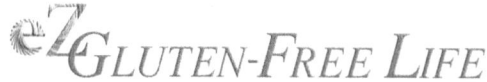
eZ GLUTEN-FREE LIFE

HAIR PRODUCTS	GF	VARIABLES
Hair Dyes:		
Avenda		Undetermined
Clairol		**GLUTEN & CC**
Eco Colors	GF	
Framesi		Undetermined
Garnier		Undetermined
Goldwell		Undetermined
Just For Men		Undetermined
L'Oreal		Undetermined
L'Oreal Professional		Undetermined
Rainbow Research	GF	
Redken		**GLUTEN**
Rene Furterer		Undetermined
Satin	GF	
Splat	GF	
Vivitone		**GLUTEN**
Xora	GF	

LIP CARE PRODUCTS	GF	VARIABLES
Alba Botanica		READ
Arbonne	GF	
Aubrey		Undetermined
Aveeno		Contains Oats
Bare Escentuals By Bare Minerals		
First Base Lip Balm	GF	
Lip Rev-er Upper	GF	

VERIFIED 2013		

COMPANY INFORMATION

No information available

http://www.clairol.com/en-US/email-us

http://www.ecocolors.net/index.cfm?pg=whatisecocolors

http://www.framesi.it/en/prodotti/scheda/73

http://www.garnierusa.com/_en/_us/services/advisor.aspx?isanswerquestion=true

http://www.goldwell-northamerica.com

http://www.combe.com/contact_thanks.asp

www.lorealparisusa.com

http://www.lorealtechnique.com/contact.aspx

▲ "We do not have prepared gluten information for our entire product line."
They do use many gluten products in production.

Henna Products

www.redken.com

http://www.folica.com/send-contact-us

http://www.developlus.com/

COMPANY INFORMATION

www.albabotanica.com

www.arbonne.com

Line to extensive. Contact Company about specific product.

www.aveeno.com

http://www.bareescentuals.com/on/demandware.store/5

▲ Which **Bare Escentuals** products are free of Wheat, Oat, Rye and/or Barley derived ingredients? While the list below shows the Wheat, Oat, Rye and Barely free products please keep in mind that these products may be made in an environment that handles Wheat, Oat, Rye and Barley derivatives.

ALWAYS READ INGREDIENTS LABELS!!!

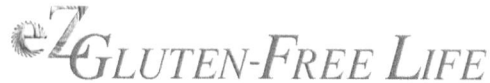

LIP CARE PRODUCTS	GF	VARIABLES
Bare Escentuals By Bare Minerals (continued):		
Makeup Remover Wipes	GF	
SPF 15 Lipgloss - Fiji	GF	
Buxom Lip Polish - all shades	GF	
Blistex	GF	
Bonnie Bell	GF	
Burst	GF	
D Votions	GF	
Definer	GF	
Frosting	GF	
Glam	GF	
Kiss This Gloss	GF	
Lites Sponge On	GF	
Boots/ Sold at Target	GF	READ **EXCEPT** **EXCEPT**
Botanic Products sold at Target		READ
Organic Body Wash	GF	
Organic Rosehip Facial	GF	
Organic Rose Toner	GF	
Burt's Bees		Undetermined
Clinique		Undetermined
Cover Girl		**GLUTEN/CC**
Dakota Free	GF	
Desert Essence Organic	GF	
Dr. Bronner	GF	
EO	GF	
Estee Lauder		Undetermined
Giovanni		Undetermined
VERIFIED 2013		

COMPANY INFORMATION

SEE MAKE UP SECTION FOR MORE DETAILS ON Bare Escentuals
ALL PRODUCTS GF
Matison & Matison 2012/2103 edition pg 536

▲ As per an email response these 2 products in the Boots line contain GLUTEN.
Dual Eye Make Up Remover contents (Triticum Vulgare Protein) wheat
No7 Moisture Drench Lipstick contains wheat germ.
As per an email response: These are the only 3 products that are GF in the Botanic
Products Line.

http://www.burtsbees.com/u/footernav/need-help/faqs.html#10
Line to extensive. Contact Company about specific product.
Company stated unable to answer question.
Owned by Maybelline
https://dakotafree.com/Category.asp?Category_Id=5
Some of the regular line and all of the Organic line is GF.
http://www.desertessence.com/faqs
www.drbronner.com
GIF certified   www.eoproducts.com
▲ Smashbox and Estee Lauder are made in the same facility.
Due to the extensive line there are "vast number of raw materials used from different
suppliers etc." Therefore they can not say if there is gluten in the products or whether go
not the products have been exposed to gluten.
Line to extensive. Contact Company about specific product.

ALWAYS READ INGREDIENTS LABELS!!!

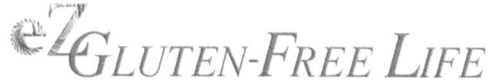

LIP CARE PRODUCTS	GF	VARIABLES
Johnson and Johnson		Undetermined
Gluten Free Beauty	GF	
Honeybee Gardens	GF	
		EXCEPT
Hugo Naturals	GF	
Jane Cosmetics		Undetermined
Jason		READ
Juice Beauty	GF	
Kissmyface		Undetermined
All Lip Shimmers	GF	
All Lip Shines	GF	
All Lip Balms	GF	
Lancome		Undetermined
MAC		Undetermined
Mill Creek		Contains Oats
Monkey Sea Monkey Doo	GF	
NARS	GF	
Neutrogena		Undetermined
Nourish	GF	
Nu Skin (Lip Products)	GF	
Oil of Olay		Undetermined
Olivina	GF	
Organique by Himalaya Herbals.		
Origins		Undetermined
VERIFIED 2013		

COMPANY INFORMATION

▲ While we perform comprehensive testing on the more common ingredients that may provide an allergic reaction such as gluten, nuts etc., unfortunately, it is impossible to test for every ingredient and we cannot guarantee that our products are gluten-free, since the source of an ingredient may change from time to time. Some of the ingredients in the product may have been purchased by us from outside distributors and we cannot say with absolute certainty that cross contamination with this ingredient did not occur at their facilities.

www.glutenfreebeauty.com

http://www.honeybeegardens.com/

▲ "I'm happy to report that our entire line, **with the exception of our hair spray,** is gluten- free. AND we are working on the hair spray to make that gluten-free as well."

http://hugonaturals.com/about-our-products

Line to extensive. Contact Company about specific product.

Read labels some of the products do contain wheat

▲ "Our Plant-based formulations come from a variety of sources and combinations of derivatives and are not screened for traces of specific allergens. We cannot guarantee that our products are gluten-free."

www.juicebeauty.com

Line to extensive. Contact Company about specific product.

www.lancome.com

Line to extensive. Contact Company about specific product.

Line to extensive. Contact Company about specific product.

www.millcreekbotanicals.com

monkeyseamonkeydoo.com (dedicated facility)

All Products GF   www.narscosmetics.com

Line to extensive. Contact Company about specific product.

www.NourishUSDA.com

www.nuskin.com

Line to extensive. Contact Company about specific product.

http://www.olivinanapavalley.com/

All GF product labeled with a green label (Shampoo has wheat).

Line to extensive. Contact Company about specific product.

ALWAYS READ INGREDIENTS LABELS!!!

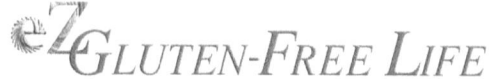

LIP CARE PRODUCTS	GF	VARIABLES
Rainbow Research	GF	
Pangea Organics	GF	
Shiseido	GF	
Tom's of Maine	GF	
		EXCEPT
Wet N Wild	GF	
		EXCEPT
Zosia Organics	GF	

Medications, over the counter drugs and supplements can have gluten.

Prescription drugs are not regulated the same as food. The FDA does not require the pharmaceutical companies to label gluten ingredients in their products. The binders in a prescription drug may contain gluten. In addition, pharmacists have no legal requirement to inform a customer if there is gluten in a product.

According to Steve Plogsted, a pharmacist at Columbus Children's Hospital and an expert on gluten free medication, "IV drugs are gluten free … and there is no chance of cross-contamination of any IV drug product." (Gluten- Free Living, Number 3, p. 50)

- For a quick and comprehensive reference use the below website, which is maintained by Steve Plogsted: http://glutenfreedrugs.com.
- You can also call the 800 number of the drug company and ask a representative if the medication has gluten. If it does have gluten please call your doctor and discuss the issue.
- The Celiac Disease Foundation website has provide the below 800 numbers, if you wish to contact the pharmaceutical companies directly.

VERIFIED 2013

COMPANY INFORMATION

▲ Some products contain colliodal oats.

http://www.pangeaorganics.com

www.sheiseido.com

All products GF except:

▲ Liquid soap & body have gluten & New antiperspirant line has gluten

Natural Moisturizing Body Wash contains wheat protein which in turn contains gluten.

http://wnwbeauty.com/

▲ Are wet n wild products gluten-free?

Most wet n wild products are gluten-free except for the following:

821A-827A Natural Blend Pressed Powder

745-749 Natural Blend Mineral Foundation and Mineral Veil

C641A MegaProtein Mascara

All other products are gluten-free.

GIG certified

Pharmaceutical Companies, 800 Phone Numbers:
  Abbott Labs - 1-800-633-9110
  Bayer (Sterling Health) 1-800-331-4536 & 1-800-332-2056
  Bristol-Meyers-Squibb 1-800-468-7746
  McNeil 1-800-962-5357
  Proctor & Gamble 1-800-395-0689
  Merck – 1-800-727-5400
  Pfizer – 800-438-1985
  Salix – 1-866-669-7597
  Eli Lilly – 1-800-545-5979

- United States National Library of Medicine: This website has supplements, vitamins, herbs, enzymes, etc listed by category and broken down by ingredients.
  http://dietarysupplements.nlm.nih.gov/dietary/specialIngred.jsp

- GFCO = Gluten-Free Certification Organization has certified several supplement companies. Since not all products produced by these companies have been certified, it is important that you review the website to confirm that what you use is GF. http://www.gfco.org/

- Celiac Disease Foundation has a detailed list of medications at the below website:
  http://www.celiac.org/index.php?option=com_content&view=article&id=44&Itemid=69

ALWAYS READ INGREDIENTS LABELS!!!

*eZ*Gluten-Free Life

MEN'S BODY CARE PRODUCTS		GF	VARIABLES
MEN'S BODY LOTIONS/MOISTURIZERS			
Gold Bond	Medicated Line- ALL	GF	
	Ultimate Line - ALL	GF	
Ecologique		GF	
EO		GF	
Eucerin			
	Skin Calming Products		**GLUTEN**
	Daily Moisturizing Products		Possible CC
	Soothing Products		Possible CC
	Intensive Repair		Possible CC
Jack Black Products			
	Cool Moisturizer Body Lotion	GF	
Kiehl Products			**GLUTEN**
Kiss My Face	Natural Moisturizers	GF	
	All Body Moisturizers	GF	
Nourish	Lotions & Polish	GF	
NuSkin	Moisturizer - All	GF	
MEN'S BODY SOAPS: BARS, SCRUBS AND WASHES			
Dr. Bonner		GF	
Dove Men	Bar Soap		Possible CC
	Body & Face Wash		Possible CC
Ecologique		GF	
EO		GF	
Gillette Body Washes		GF	
Kiehl Products			**GLUTEN**
Kiss My Face	Olive Bars -ALL	GF	
	Shower Gels -ALL	GF	
	Organic Foaming Soap	GF	**EXCEPT**
NuSkin	All Soaps & Cleansers	GF	
Olay Pro X (Gillette)		GF	

VERIFIED 2013

COMPANY INFORMATION

http://goldbond.com/

http:/goldbond.com/

http://formulacorp.com/personal-care/

www.eoproducts.com

Contain Oats

Contains no gluten ingredients but has not been tested for CC.

Formulas are changed often. Read Labels.

▲ Jack Black website Click "Ways To Shop" Ribbon. Click gluten-free products.

▲ The line uses gluten in many products with extensive chemical names for gluten.
   Vitamin E is made with cereal germ oil (gluten) READ LABELS.

Call 1-877-712-9992

http://www.nourishusda.com/

www.nuskin.com

http://www.drbronner.com/

Contains no gluten ingredients -has not been tested for CC.

Contains no gluten ingredients -has not been tested for CC.

http://formulacorp.com/personal-care/

www.eoproducts.com

All Gillette Body Wash Products are GF

▲ The line uses gluten in many products with extensive chemical names for gluten.
   Vitamin E is made with cereal germ oil (gluten) READ LABELS.

Call 1-877-712-9992

Castile Peace Soap Line

www.nuskin.com

http://www.olay.com/skin-care-products/OlayPro-X

All Olay Pro X Products are Gluten Free

ALWAYS READ INGREDIENTS LABELS!!!

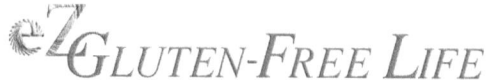
EZ GLUTEN-FREE LIFE

MEN'S BODY CARE PRODUCTS		GF	VARIABLES
MEN'S BODY SOAPS: BARS, SCRUBS AND WASHES			
Origins			Undetermined
	Skin Diver® Body Wash		Undetermined
	Skin Diver® Body Soap		Undetermined
	Skin Diver® Body Scrub		Undetermined
Shiseido	Cleansing Foam	GF	
	Deep Cleansing Scrub	GF	
Tom's of Maine	Bar Soap	GF	
	Washes		**GLUTEN**
Z Zegna	Body Wash		**GLUTEN**

Most condoms use **corn starch** in the packaging. Casein, a milk protein, is often used as an emulsifier or binding agent in condoms. Gluten (wheat, barley, rye or oats)

CONDOMS	GF/Gluten GF=Gluten-free	DF/ Contains Corn DF=Dairy-free and Vegan	Latex
Beyond Seven®	GF	DF/ Contains Corn	Latex
Condomi®	Undetermined	DF/Undetermined	Non Latex
Durex Latex®			Latex
Natural Rubber Latex	Undetermined	Dairy/Undetermined	Latex
Durex® Non-latex			Non Latex
Durex Avanti	Undetermined	DF/Undetermined	Non Latex
Real Fell	Undetermined	DF/Undetermined	Non Latex
Fetherlite Ultra	Undetermined	DF/Undetermined	Non Latex
Fetherlite Deluxe	Undetermined	DF/Undetermined	Non Latex
GLYDE®	GF	DF/Undetermined	Non Latex
Kimono®	GF	DF/Undetermined	Latex
Okamoto Crown®	GF	DF/Undetermined	Latex
Protex®	Undetermined	Undetermined	Latex
Sir Richard's®	GF	DF/ Contains Corn	Latex

VERIFIED 2013

COMPANY INFORMATION

Company did not respond to requests for information. 1-800-ORIGINS

Company did not respond to requests for information. 1-800-ORIGINS

Company did not respond to requests for information. 1-800-ORIGINS

Company did not respond to requests for information. 1-800-ORIGINS

www.shiseido.com

www.shiseido.com

www.tomsofmaine.com

www.zzegna.com

COMPANY INFORMATION

Okamoto USA Inc (Contains corn)

http://www.condomicondoms.org/

http://www.durex.com/en-GB/Products/condoms/Pages/Durex-SelectFlavours.aspx#5

▲ Natural Rubber latex condoms are suitable for vegetarians; they contain an ingredient called casein (milk derivative) but no other animal related products.

▲ Our non- latex condom (Durex Avanti, Real Feel, Fetherlite Ultra and Deluxe) are free of animal-derived products and suitable for vegans.

http://www.glydeamerica.com/safer-sex-faq/

http://www.kimono-condoms.com/condom_questions.htm#7c

Okamoto USA Inc (Contains corn)

Company did not respond to my requests for information.

1-855-303-7722

ALWAYS READ INGREDIENTS LABELS!!!

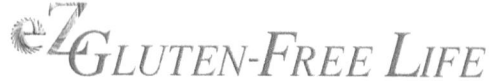

MEN'S BODY CARE PRODUCTS			
CONDOMS	**GF/Gluten** *GF=Gluten-free*	**DF/ Contains Corn** *DF=Dairy-free* *and Vegan*	**Latex**
Skyn® by Lifestyle®	Undetermined	Undetermined	Non Latex
Original	Undetermined	Undetermined	Non Latex
Extra Lubricated	Undetermined	Undetermined	Non Latex
Large	Undetermined	Undetermined	Non Latex
Trojan® Products:			
Armor®	No gluten added	Dairy/Contains Corn	Latex
Charged™ by Trojan®	No gluten added	Dairy/ Contains Corn	Latex
Bareskin®	No gluten added	READ/Contains Corn	Latex
Ecstasy™ by Trojan®	No gluten added	Dairy/Contains Corn	Latex
Enz®	No gluten added	Dairy/Contains Corn	Latex
Extended by Trojan®	No gluten added	Dairy/Contains Corn	Latex
Fire & Ice®	No gluten added	Dairy/Contains Corn	Latex
Her Pleasure™ by Trojan®	No gluten added	Dairy/Contains Corn	Latex
Magnum®	No gluten added	Dairy/Contains Corn	Latex
NaturaLamb®	No gluten added	DF/Contains Corn	Non Latex
Pleasures®	No gluten added	Dairy/Contains Corn	Latex
Sensitivity®	No gluten added	Dairy/Contains Corn	Latex
Stimulation®	No gluten added	Dairy/Contains Corn	Latex
Supra®	No gluten added	Dairy/ Contains Corn	Non Latex
Thintensity®	No gluten added	READ/Contains Corn	Latex
Ultra Ribbed Lubricated by Trojan®	No gluten added	Dairy/ Contains Corn	Latex
Personal Lubricants:			
Astroglide® Gel	Undetermined	Undetermined	
Astroglide® Liquid	Undetermined	Undetermined	
Astroglide® Gel	Undetermined	Undetermined	
Astroglide® X Silicone	Undetermined	Undetermined	
Astroglide® Natural	Undetermined	Undetermined	

VERIFIED 2013

COMPANY INFORMATION

http://www.lifestyles.com/condom-faqs/#qC10
Company did not respond to my requests for information.
Company did not respond to my requests for information.
Company did not respond to my requests for information.
▲ 1-877-320-3075 Church and Dwight Company
Casein, which is a dairy by-product, is in all condoms with a TT lot code.
Trojan® Thintensity® and Trojan® Bareskin® Condoms with lot codes beginning with CZ or DA, do not contain casein. We do not knowingly include gluten in any of our condoms.
www.churchwright.com

http://www.astroglide.com/products/astroglidegel.aspx
Company did not respond to my requests for information.
Company did not respond to my requests for information.
Company did not respond to my requests for information.
Company did not respond to my requests for information.

ALWAYS READ INGREDIENTS LABELS!!!

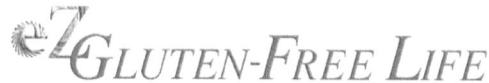

MEN'S BODY CARE PRODUCTS CONDOMS	GF/Gluten *GF=Gluten-free*	DF/ Contains Corn *DF=Dairy-free and Vegan*	Latex
Personal Lubricants (continued):			
Astroglide® Gel (continued)	Undetermined	Undetermined	
Glycerin & Paraben Free	Undetermined	Undetermined	
Sensual Strawberry	Undetermined	Undetermined	
Astroglide® Warming	Undetermined	Undetermined	
Blossom Organic			
Equate®	Undetermined	Undetermined	
ID Glide®	Undetermined	Undetermined	
K-Y®	Undetermined	Undetermined	
Liquid Silk™	Undetermined	Undetermined	
Maximus™	Undetermined	Undetermined	
Passion Lubes®	Undetermined	Undetermined	

MEN'S BODY CARE PRODUCTS		GF	VARIABLES
MEN'S DEODORANT/ANTIPERSPIRANT			
Axe Effect Deodorant			Undetermined
Dove Men	Antiperspirants		Possible CC
	Deodorants		Possible CC
EO	Deodorants	GF	
Honeybee Gardens For Men			
	Deodorant Powder	GF	
Irish Spring®			Possible CC
Kiehl Products	Deodorant/Antiperspirants		**GLUTEN**
Kiss My Face	All Liquid Rock Deodorant	GF	
Nourish	Deodorant	GF	
Speed Stick® Regular			Possible CC
Speed Stick®24/7®			Possible CC
Speed Stick®Musk			Possible CC
VERIFIED 2013			

COMPANY INFORMATION

http://www.astroglide.com/products/astroglidegel.aspx
Company did not respond to my requests for information.
Company did not respond to my requests for information.
Company did not respond to my requests for information.

No contact information
Company did not respond to my requests for information.
Company did not respond to my requests for information.
Company did not respond to my requests for information.
Company did not respond to my requests for information.
No contact information http://www.passionlubes.com/

COMPANY INFORMATION

http://www.theaxeeffect.com/faq.html
Contains no gluten ingredients -has not been tested for CC.
Contains no gluten ingredients -has not been tested for CC.
www.eoproducts.com

http://www.honeybeegardens.com/
Contains no gluten ingredients -has not been tested.
▲ The line uses gluten in many products with extensive chemical names for gluten.
   Vitamin E is made with cereal germ oil (gluten) READ LABELS.
1-877-712-9992
http://www.nourishusda.com/
Contains no gluten ingredients -has not been tested for CC.
Contains no gluten ingredients -has not been tested for CC.
Contains no gluten ingredients -has not been tested for CC.

ALWAYS READ INGREDIENTS LABELS!!!

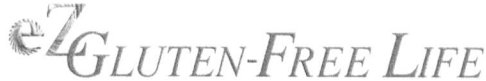

MEN'S BODY CARE PRODUCTS	GF	VARIABLES
MEN'S DEODORANT/ANTIPERSPIRANT		
Speed Stick®OceanSurf® Clear		Possible CC
Speed Stick®Power®		Possible CC
Speed Stick®StainGuard®		Possible CC
Tom's of Maine Deodorants		Possible CC
Antiperspirants - ALL		**GLUTEN**
Z Zegna Deodorant Stick		**GLUTEN**
FACE MOISTURIZIERS		
A*Men by Thierry Mugler		GF
Arbonne (RE Advanced)		
Facial Moisturizer SPF20	GF	
Ahava	GF	**EXCEPT**
Dr Dennis Gross Skincare	GF	**EXCEPT**
Jack Black Products		
Double-Duty Face Moisturizer	GF	
Protein Booster Eye Rescue	GF	
Kiss My Face		
Brightening Day Crème	GF	
Eyewitness Eye Repair Crème	GF	**EXCEPT**
Neutrogena		
Oil-Free Moisturizer SPF 30		Possible CC
Age-Fighter Face w SPF 15	GF	
Triple Protection Face Lotion w SPF 20	GF	
NuSkin Moisturizer - All	GF	
Olay Pro X (Gillette)	GF	
Origins - Save The Face®		
Moisturizer		Undetermined
Shiseido Hydrating Lotion	GF	
Moisturizing Emulsion	GF	

VERIFIED 2013

COMPANY INFORMATION

Contains no gluten ingredients -has not been tested for CC.
Contains no gluten ingredients -has not been tested for CC.
Contains no gluten ingredients -has not been tested for CC.
www.tomsofmaine.com

www.zzegna.com

1-866-868-4537

www.arbonne.com
www.ahavaus.com
Night Replenisher N/D
▲ All in One Facial Cleanser with Toner contains Avena Sativa (Oat) Kernel Extract
Hydrating Body Emulsion, Purifying Bath Crystals and Creamy Cleansing Polish contain Colloidal Oatmeal 1-888-830-7546

▲ http://www.getjackblack.com/glutenfree.aspx
▲ Jack Black website click "Ways To Shop" Ribbon. Click gluten-free products.
1-877-712-9992
Face Moisturizer
C The Change Serum
So Refined
Vitamin E is made with cereal germ oil (gluten) READ LABELS.
1-800-582-4048
Contains no gluten but has not yet been tested.

www.nuskin.com
http://www.olay.com/skin-care-products/OlayPro-X
All Olay Pro X Products are Gluten Free

Company did not respond to requests for information. 1-800-ORIGINS
www.shiseido.com

ALWAYS READ INGREDIENTS LABELS!!!

eZGLUTEN-FREE LIFE

MEN'S BODY CARE PRODUCTS		GF	VARIABLES
FACE MOISTURIZIERS			
Shiseido: Special Face Care			
	Deep Wrinkle Corrector	GF	
	Eye Soother	GF	
	Total Revitalizer	GF	
	Energizing Formula	GF	
Yve Saint Laurent			**GLUTEN**
FACE WASHERS/SCRUBS			
Arbonne (RE Advanced)		GF	
Ahava		GF	
Jack Black Products			
	DIY Power Peel Multi-Acid	GF	
	Resurface Pads		
	Pure Clean Daily Face Cleaner	GF	
Kiehl Products			**GLUTEN**
Kiss My Face	Pore Shrink Cleansing Mask	GF	**EXCEPT**
	Shea Soy Facial Bar	GF	
	Start Up Exfoliating Face Wash	GF	
Neutrogena	Men®Razor Defense® Face Scrub	GF	
	Men®Skin Clearing Acne Wash	GF	
Olay Pro X (Gillette)		GF	
FOOT CARE PRODUCTS			
Gold Bond	Medicated Line - All	GF	
	Ultimate Line - All	GF	
Kiehl Products			**GLUTEN**
HAIR PRODUCTS			
100% Pure		GF	
365 Premium Body Care		GF	
Alterna (Bamboo Line)		GF	
			EXCEPT
Arbonne		GF	
Aubrey			**READ LABELS**
Aveeno			Contains Oats
Aveda			**READ/CC**
VERIFIED 2013			

COMPANY INFORMATION

www.shiseido.com

Company suggests reading ingredient list which uses FDA approved names for gluten.

www.arbonne.com

www.ahavaus.com

▲ http://www.getjackblack.com/glutenfree.aspx

▲ Jack Black website click "Ways To Shop" Ribbon. Click gluten-free products.

▲ The line uses gluten in many products with extensive chemical names for gluten.
Vitamin E is made with cereal germ oil (gluten) READ LABELS.

1-877-712-9992

Clean For A Day

1-800-582-4048

http://www.olay.com/skin-care-products/OlayPro-X

http://goldbond.com/

http://goldbond.com/

▲ The line uses gluten in many products with extensive chemical names for gluten.
Vitamin E is made with cereal germ oil (gluten) READ LABELS.

www.alterna.com

Kendi Oil has wheat

www.arbonne.com

www.aubrey.com

www.aveeno.com

▲ 1-888-424-7707 Aveda states that some of the products may be made without gluten

ALWAYS READ INGREDIENTS LABELS!!!

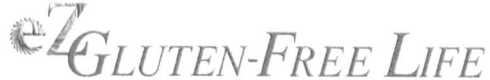

Gluten-Free Life

MEN'S BODY CARE PRODUCTS	GF	VARIABLES
HAIR PRODUCTS		
BedHead by TIGI		**READ**
Catwalk by TIGI		**GLUTEN**
Clairol		**GLUTEN/CC**
Clinique		Undetermined
Desert Essences Organic	GF	**READ**
Desert Essences Non Organic		Undetermined
Dove Men Hair Care-ALL Products	GF	**READ**
Dr. Bronner - ALL Products	GF	
Ecologique	GF	
Shampoo & Conditioner		
EO	GF	
Head & Shoulders (Gillette)	GF	
ALL Products		
Honeybee Gardens	GF	
		EXCEPT
Hugo Natural	GF	
Just For Men Hair Dye		**GLUTEN**
Beard & Hair Dye		
Kiehl Products		**GLUTEN**
Matrix		Undetermined
Method	GF	
Mill Creek		Contains Oats
Morroco Method	GF	
Neutrogena	GF	
S factor by TIGI		**GLUTEN**
VERIFIED 2013		

COMPANY INFORMATION

▲ TIGI sent an email listing the gluten-free products their brands have. The only line is BedHead. Email stated that though some products are GF they cannot guarantee cross contaminated. Please call 800-259-8596 for an extensive list of BedHead GF products.

▲ TIGI states that their only gluten-free line is BedHead.

www.clariol.com

Line too extensive. Contact company about specific product. www.clinique.com

Only the organic line is 100% GF

http://www.desertessence.com/faqs

Contains no gluten ingredients -has not been tested for CC.

www.drbonner.com

http://formulacorp.com/personal-care/

www.eoproducts.com

*Head & Shoulders (US Shampoos, 2in1's and Conditioners)

All USA/CA Head & Shoulders products are GF Skin Care

http://www.honeybeegardens.com/

Hairspray has gluten! All other products GF.

The products may have oats that are GF.

Contains wheat: 1-800-431-2610

The line uses gluten in many products with extensive chemical names for gluten.

Read labels to be sure.

▲ http://methodhome.com/support/faqs/

"Thanks so much for taking the time to write to us and for your interest in method. Actually, all of our products are gluten free and safe for those with Celiac's disease. We don't use wheat or gluten in any of our ingredients."

www.millcreekbotanicals.com

https://morroccomethod.com/

Line too extensive to give details.

▲ TIGI states that their only gluten-free line is BedHead.

ALWAYS READ INGREDIENTS LABELS!!!

ℰ𝒵 GLUTEN-FREE LIFE

MEN'S BODY CARE PRODUCTS	GF	VARIABLES
HAIR PRODUCTS		
TIGI Products		**GLUTEN**
Organix Beauty Pure & Simple	GF	
		EXCEPT
Pureology Products		**GLUTEN**
Sophyto	GF	
Sauve		**GLUTEN/CC**
Unite		**GLUTEN/CC**
Weleda		**GLUTEN/CC**
Wen By Chaz Dean		**GLUTEN**
Z Zegna		
Hair Products		Contains Oats
LIP CARE		
Blistex	GF	
Lip balms, sticks		
Dr. Bonner		
Lip balms, sticks	GF	
EO		
Lip balms, sticks	GF	
Shea Butter & Vitamin E	GF	
Vanilla & Lavender	GF	
Jack Black Products		
Intensive Lip Therapy Balm	GF	
Black Tea & Blackberry	GF	
Grapefruit & Ginger	GF	
Lemon & Chamomile	GF	
Mango and Mandarin	GF	
Natural Mint & Shea Butter	GF	
Coconut Pineapple SPF 15	GF	
Kiehl Products		**GLUTEN**
Strawberry SPF 15	GF	
Treatment Lip Balm SPF 15	GF	
VERIFIED 2013		

COMPANY INFORMATION

▲ TIGI sent an email listing the gluten-free products their brands have. The only line is BedHead. Email stated that though some products are GF they cannot guarantee cross contaminated. Please call 800-259-8596 for an extensive list of BedHead GF products.

www.organixhair.com/content/faq

Biotin and Collagen Line which contains Hydrolyzed Wheat Protein

Read labels as per email

Certified GF www.sophyto.com

▲ Via email I communicated with the company who claimed their products is gluten free yet I found WHEAT PROTEIN in several of their products.

usa.weleda.com

Contains wheat protein

www.zzegna.com

All Blistex products are GF

http://www.drbronner.com/

www.eoproducts.com

▲ Jack Black website click "Ways To Shop" Ribbon. Click gluten-free products.

▲ The line uses gluten in many products with extensive chemical names for gluten. Vitamin E is made with cereal germ oil (gluten) READ LABELS.

ALWAYS READ INGREDIENTS LABELS!!!

MEN'S BODY CARE PRODUCTS	GF	VARIABLES
LIP CARE		
Kiss My Face		**EXCEPT**
Lip Balms: Only Below Flavors	GF	
Sliced Peach SPF 15	GF	
Cranberry Orange SPF 15	GF	
Ginger Mango SPF 15	GF	
Vanilla Honey SPF 15	GF	
SHAVING PRODUCTS		
AFTER SHAVE		
Arbonne (RE Advanced)		
Post Shave Balm	GF	
Afta by Colgate		Possible CC
Ahava	GF	**EXCEPT**
Honeybee Gardens	GF	
Kiehl Products		**GLUTEN**
L'Occitane		**READ**
Nivea (Beiersdorf)		Undetermined
Origins - Fire Fighter®		Undetermined
Yve Saint Laurent		**GLUTEN**
Z Zegna		
After Shave		**GLUTEN**
RAZOR PRODUCTS		
Fusion by Gillette		
LubriStrips for razors	GF	
VERIFIED 2013		

COMPANY INFORMATION

All other Lip Balms
Call 1-877-712-9992

www.arbonne.com

▲ "...we do not intentionally add gluten to any of our other products. Though we obtain our ingredients from reliable and trusted suppliers who maintain our high standards for safety, quality, and efficacy, we cannot guarantee that the ingredients used have not come in contact with any gluten."

www.ahavaus.com
Night Replenisher N/D
Mineral Foot Cream
The make-up line
The sun care line

http://www.honeybeegardens.com/

▲ The line uses gluten in many products with extensive chemical names for gluten. Vitamin E is made with cereal germ oil (gluten) READ LABELS.

▲ We do have products that contain wheat proteins but no gluten this is due to the fact that the gluten is separated out and removed from the products. After the process is complete tests are done to ensure that the wheat proteins used "do not show any peak of native gluten".

▲ The company suggests that, "If you have concerns about gluten and its derivatives, we recommend avoiding all products with the ingredients wheat, barley or rye."

Company did not respond to my requests for information. 1-800-ORIGINS

Company suggests reading ingredient list which uses FDA approved names for gluten.

www.zzegna.com

www.gillette.com

ALWAYS READ INGREDIENTS LABELS!!!

eZ GLUTEN-FREE LIFE

MEN'S BODY CARE PRODUCTS	GF	VARIABLES
SHAVING GEL/CREAMS		
Arbonne (RE Advanced)		
Shave Gel	GF	
Ahava	GF	**EXCEPT**
Dr. Bonner		
Shaving Gel	GF	
EO	GF	
Splash, Foam & Cream		
Fusion Products by Gillette		
Clear Pro Glide Shaving Gel	GF	
HydraGel Cooling	GF	
Irritation Defense Gel	GF	
Moisturizing	GF	
Pure & Sensitive	GF	
Gillette Company		
Pre Shave Formulas		Undetermined
Sensitive Shave Foam		Undetermined
Shave Gel		Undetermined
Extra Comfort		Undetermined
Moisturizing		Undetermined
Shaving Therapy		
Kiehl Products		**GLUTEN**
Kiss My Face		
Peaches & Créme	GF	READ
Fragrance Free		
Cool Mint		**EXCEPT**
Key Lime		
Patchouli		
Lavender & Shea		
VERIFIED 2013		

COMPANY INFORMATION

www.arbonne.com

www.ahavaus.com
Night Replenisher N/D
Mineral Foot Cream
The make-up line
The sun care line
http://www.drbronner.com/

www.eoproducts.com

www.gillette.com

▲ www.gillette.com
Line is too Extensive. Contact company about specific product.
Line is too Extensive. Contact company about specific product.
Line is too Extensive. Contact company about specific product.
Line is too Extensive. Contact company about specific product.
Line is too Extensive. Contact company about specific product.
"Our plant-based formulations come from a variety of sources and combinations of derivatives and are not screened for allergens. We cannot guarantee that our products are gluten-free."
▲ The line uses gluten in many products with extensive chemical names for gluten.
   Vitamin E is made with cereal germ oil (gluten) READ LABELS.

Call Kiss My Face for a detailed list of their GF items.
1-877-712-9992
Green Tea Bamboo & Pomegranate Grapefruit Shave Products

ALWAYS READ INGREDIENTS LABELS!!!

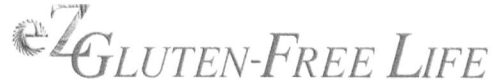

MEN'S BODY CARE PRODUCTS	GF	VARIABLES
SHAVING GEL/CREAMS		
L'Occitane		READ
Nivea (Beiersdorf)		Undetermined
Neutrogena		
Post Shave Lotion	GF	
Face Scrub	GF	
Men® Sensitive Skin		
Shave Cream	GF	
Post Shave Lotion	GF	
Oil-Free Moisturizer w SPF30		Possible CC
Men® Skin Clearing	GF	
Origins		
Blade Runner®		Undetermined
Easy Slider®		Undetermined
Personna Shaving Cream	GF	READ
Schick Shaving Cream	GF	READ
Shiseido	GF	
Skintimate Shaving Cream	GF	READ
Wilkinson Sword Shaving Cream	GF	READ

VERIFIED 2013

COMPANY INFORMATION

▲ We do have products that contain wheat proteins but no gluten – this is due to the fact that the gluten is separated out and removed from the products. After the process is complete tests are done to ensure that the wheat proteins used "do not show any peak of native gluten".

The company suggests that, "If you have concerns about gluten and its derivatives, we recommend avoiding all products with the ingredients wheat, barley or rye." 1-800-582-4048

Contains no gluten but has not yet been tested for CC.

Company did not respond to my requests for information. 1-800-ORIGINS
Company did not respond to my requests for information. 1-800-ORIGINS

"None of our razors or shaving gel and creams contain gluten in any form." Energizer Personal Care.
"None of our razors or shaving gel and creams contain gluten in any form." Energizer Personal Care.
www.shiseido.com
"None of our razors or shaving gel and creams contain gluten in any form." Energizer Personal Care.
"None of our razors or shaving gel and creams contain gluten in any form." Energizer Personal Care.

ALWAYS READ INGREDIENTS LABELS!!!

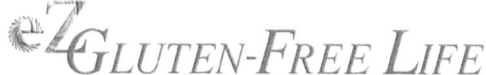

GLUTEN-FREE LIFE

Please note that the larger companies and those owned by large corporations are often unable to answer whether or not there is gluten or if they are exposed to cross contamination because of the size of the line. The vast number of suppliers they use and the fact that the manufacturing plants often produce products with gluten right next to products without gluten. Please contact the company direct for further information.

MEN'S BODY CARE PRODUCTS	VARIABLES
Aramis	Undetermined
Burts Bees	Undetermined
Calvin Klein	Undetermined
Clinque Men's	Undetermined
Dolce & Gabanna	Undetermined
Lab Series	Undetermined
Neutrogena	Undetermined
Philosophy	Undetermined
Polo	Undetermined
Ralph Lauren	Undetermined
The Art of Shaving	Undetermined
Many Men's Skin Care and Perfume Lines are unprepared to answer the question as to whether there is gluten in the products. Perfume Lines do not always clearly label wheat, barley or rye product in the ingredients list.	
Boss (Hugo Boss)	Undetermined
Cartier	Undetermined
Gucci	Undetermined
Hermes	Undetermined
Jaipur	Undetermined
Jean Paul Gaulteir	Undetermined
Jo Malone	Undetermined
John Varvatos	Undetermined
MontBlanc	Undetermined
Tom Ford	Undetermined
Versace	Undetermined
Vince Camuto	Undetermined
VERIFIED 2013	

COMPANY INFORMATION

Owned by Estee Lauder, "Due to the extensive line there are "vast number of raw materials used from different suppliers, etc."

Line is too Extensive. Contact company about specific product.

Line is too Extensive. Contact company about specific product.

1-866-214-6694

www.clinque.com

Line is too Extensive. Contact company about specific product.

Owned by P&G Line too Extensive. Contact company about specific products.

Line is too Extensive. Contact company about specific product.

Line is too Extensive. Contact company about specific product.

Company requests that you read labels and discuss questions with doctor.

Line is too Extensive. Contact company about specific product.

Line is too Extensive. Contact company about specific product.

Line is too Extensive. Contact company about specific product.

Company was unable to answer the question.

Company was unable to answer the question.

Company was unable to answer the question.

Company was unable to answer the question.

Company was unable to answer the question.

Company was unable to answer the question.

Company was unable to answer the question.

Company was unable to answer the question.

Company was unable to answer the question.

Company was unable to answer the question.

Company was unable to answer the question.

Company was unable to answer the question.

ALWAYS READ INGREDIENTS LABELS!!!

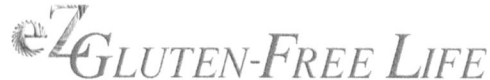

MEN'S BODY CARE PRODUCTS	ITEM NAME
MEN'S BRANDS	
Perfume/Cologne Lines do not always label barley or rye products in the ingredients list.	
Companies did not respond to my requests for information.	
Acqua di Parma	deodorant, after shave
Anthony Logistics	face, after shave, shave
B The Product	hair
Billy Jealousy	body, hair, face, shave, after shave
Boucheron	deodorant, face
BVLGARI	cologne
ClarinsMen	body lotion, deodorant, face, after shave, shave
Doctor T's Supergoob	sunscreen
English Laundry	face,hair
HiM Hanae Mori	after shave
J Paul	cologne
Mënaji	face, after shave
Sisley	deodorant, face
Tela Beauty Organics	hair
Viktor & Rolf	cologne
Z Zegra	after shave

NAIL PRODUCTS	GF	VARIABLES
Bonnie Bell	GF	
Nail Lacquers	GF	
Cutex	GF	
Dakota Free	GF	
Honeybee Gardens	GF	
		EXCEPT
Kiss (Nail Products)	GF	
VERIFIED 2013		

COMPANY INFORMATION

Company did not respond to my requests for information.
Company did not respond to my requests for information.
Company did not respond to my requests for information.
Company did not respond to my requests for information.
Company did not respond to my requests for information.
Company did not respond to my requests for information.
Company did not respond to my requests for information.

Company did not respond to my requests for information.
Company did not respond to my requests for information.
Company did not respond to my requests for information.
Company did not respond to my requests for information.
Company did not respond to my requests for information.
Company did not respond to my requests for information.
Company did not respond to my requests for information.
Company did not respond to my requests for information.
Company did not respond to my requests for information.

COMPANY INFORMATION
As per Matison & Matison 2012/2013 edition pg 520

ALL PRODUCTS GF
www.dakotafree.com
www.honeybeegardens.com
▲ "I'm happy to report that our entire line, with the exception of our hair spray, is gluten-free. AND we are working on the hair spray to make that gluten-free as well."
www.kissusa.com
▲ Nail products such as glue, fakeon nails, nail paint, stickers & jewelry.

ALWAYS READ INGREDIENTS LABELS!!!

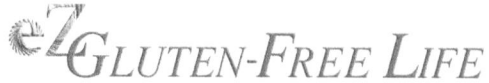

NAIL PRODUCTS	GF	VARIABLES
La Fresh Wipes	GF	
NARS	GF	
Onyx	GF	**EXCEPT**
OPI		READ
		GLUTEN
Peacekeeper		Undetermined
Pink (Nail products for girls)	GF	
Sally Hansen		READ
		Undetermined
Wet N Wild	GF	**EXCEPT**
VERIFIED 2013		

COMPANY INFORMATION

▲ Have all natural ingredients and are gluten-free. They are great for traveling or for someone on the go. DOES NOT CARRY POLISH.
Products include: Acetone-Free Nail Polisher Remover

www.nars.com (Has base coat, top coat & polish)

Hoof Foot Care

www.opi.com verfied 5/2012

▲ The following OPI products contain hydrolyzed wheat and/or oat protein, which may have traces of gluten.

These products should definitely be avoided by anyone with gluten sensitivity:
Acrylic Nail Base Coat
Feet – Clear Matte nail strengthener
Start to Finish basecoat, topcoat, and nail strengthener
Start to Finish, Formaldehyde Free Formula

Nail Envy, Original
Nail Envy, Matte
Nail Envy, Maintenance
Nail Envy, Dry & Brittle
Nail Envy, Sensitive & Peeling
Nail Envy, Soft & Thin

Nail Envy: Nail Strengthener
Nail Envy, Cool Pink (limited distribution)
Nail Envy, Warm Peach (limited distribution
Nicole by OPI Strengthener Plus
Nic's Stics – Tough Gir

At this time, all other currently manufactured OPI products should contain no gluten except. See attached statement.

http://www.iamapeacekeeper.com/

www.kissusa.com, email response 4/2012

▲ Nail products such as glue, fakeon nails, nail paint, stickers & jewelry.

http://www.sallyhansen.com

▲ "As required by law, each product's package, insert or hang-tag exhibits a complete list of its ingredients. If the words "gluten," "wheat", "barley", "rye", or "oat" are absent from that ingredient listing, then the product was not formulated to include gluten. For your convenience, a list of specific cosmetics ingredients derived from these grain sources is enclosed." This list contains over 200 cosmetic ingredients containing gluten. See attached ingredients list.

http://wnwbeauty.com/

▲ Are wet n wild products gluten-free?
Most wet n wild products are gluten-free except for the following:
821A-827A Natural Blend Pressed Powder. 745-749 Natural Blend Mineral Foundation and Mineral Veil. C641A MegaProtein Mascara. All other products are gluten-free.

ALWAYS READ INGREDIENTS LABELS!!!

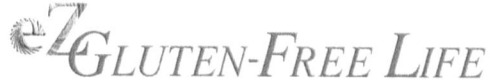

PERSONAL HYGIENE PRODUCTS	GF	VARIABLES
La Fresh Wipes: Have all natural ingredients and gluten-free.	GF	
Vagisil Creams		
Regular Strength	GF	
Maximum Strength	GF	
Kimberly Clark: As of 2012		
Adult Hygiene		
Depends	GF	
Poise	GF	**EXCEPT**
Feminine Hygiene		
Kotex	GF	
Kimberly Clark: As of 2012		
Paper Products		
Kleenex (All Kleenex products)	GF	
Cottonelle (Bathroom wipes)	GF	
Scotts	GF	
Viva	GF	
VERIFIED 2013		

COMPANY INFORMATION

▲ They are great for traveling or for someone on the go.
Products include:
Waterproof Make-up Remover
Oil-free Face Cleanser
Instant Body Soother
Healthy Hand Sanitizer
Acetone-Free Nail Polisher Remover
Travel-Lite Easy Packets:
Deodorant for Men and Women, Feminine Wipes, Hydrating Lotion, Sunscreen, Len's Cleaner, Screen Cleaners & Shoe Shine
1-800-431-2610

Thanks for your e-mail to Kimberly-Clark.

▲ Kimberly-Clark consumer products do not contain wheat, rye, barley, spelt, triticale, kamut or farina. Certain Kimberly-Clark products do contain oats. The only Kimberly-Clark products containing oats are HUGGIES® Soft Skin products.

ALWAYS READ INGREDIENTS LABELS!!!

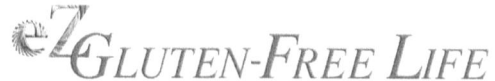

PERSONAL HYGIENE PRODUCTS	GF	VARIABLES
Health Care & Professional Products see:		
Wet Ones (Wipes)		Undetermined
Feminine Hygiene Products:		
Always	GF	
Tampax	GF	
Natracare	GF	
Playtex		Undetermined
		READ
Seventh Generation		READ

VERIFIED 2013

COMPANY INFORMATION

http://www.kimberly-clark.com/brands/kc_healthcare.aspx
http://www.kimberly-clark.com/brands/kc_professional.aspx

▲ I received the same response over the phone. We understand your concern about ensuring the products you are using do not contain gluten. With regard to our line of sun care products, although we do not use wheat protein or wheat derived oils in our product formulations, we cannot certify that our facilities are gluten free. In addition, the plant origin of some ingredients may vary, making Gluten Free Certification difficult. We regret we are not able to suggest a product that meets your needs at this time. For specific information on this ingredient as well as other sun care and cosmetic product ingredients, please visit www.cosmeticsinfo.org.

▲ We do not use gluten in the manufacture of Always Pads, Liners, Wipes or Tampax tampons.

▲ "I am happy to let you know that all Natracare products are Gluten Free."

▲ With regard to our line of Playtex products, although we do not use wheat protein or wheat derived oils in our product formulations, we cannot certify that our facilities are gluten free. In addition, the plant origin of some ingredients may vary, making Gluten Free Certification difficult. We regret we are not able to suggest a product that meets your needs at this time. For specific information on this ingredient as well as other sun care and cosmetic product ingredients, please visit www.cosmeticsinfo.org.

▲ Does Seventh Generation have *gluten* in their cleaning products?

Seventh Generation does not test any of our products for the presence of *gluten*; therefore, we cannot guarantee that any of products are *gluten* free. "However, our products are comprised of ingredients that are naturally gluten-free; and ingredients that may potentially be derived from gluten-containing plant sources (wheat, rye, barley, and oats) are rendered *gluten* free through their extensive processing. Seventh Generation products are not intended for consumption, which should eliminate any concern of *gluten* entering your digestive system; however, we understand that there are some individuals with severe forms of Celiac Disease who cannot touch *gluten*. Please consult your physician if you are concerned about which cleaning and personal care products might be right for you."

ALWAYS READ INGREDIENTS LABELS!!!

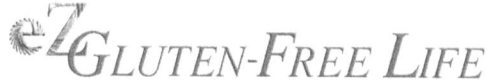

SUNSCREEN PRODUCTS	GF	VARIABLES
Alba Botanica		Undetermined
All Terrain	GF	
Arbonne	GF	
Aveeno		Contains Oats
Baby Blanket		
Badger	GF	READ
Banana Boat		Undetermined
Burt's Bees		Undetermined
Clinique		Undetermined
California Baby	GF	
Coppertone	GF	
Water Babies& Kids Pure & Simple	GF	
UltraGuard SPF 30	GF	
Solacane	GF	
Dakota Free	GF	
Desert Essences Organics	GF	
Eco	GF	
VERIFIED 2013		

COMPANY INFORMATION

www.albabotanica.com

▲ "Our plant-based formulations come from a variety of sources and combinations of derivatives and are not screened for traces of specific allergens. We cannot guarantee that our products are gluten-free."

www.allterrain.com

www.arbonne.com

www.aveeno.com

http://www.babyblanketsuncare.com/thanks.htm

http://www.badgerbalm.com/t-faq.aspx

▲ I have allergies to Peanuts and Gluten. Are Badger Products safe for me to use? "Badger products contain no peanuts, peanut oils, wheat or gluten. However, the facility that fills our lip balms also uses wheat amino acids and wheat protein, so there is the possibility of cross-contamination. Our facility is not certified as "gluten free", but uses no wheat or gluten containing ingredients.

▲ "We understand your concern about ensuring the products you are using do not contain gluten. With regard to our line of sun care products, although we do not use wheat protein or wheat derived oils in our product formulations, we cannot certify that our facilities are gluten free. In addition, the plant origin of some ingredients may vary, making Gluten Free Certification difficult. We regret we are not able to suggest a product that meets your needs at this time. For specific information on this ingredient as well as other sun care and cosmetic product ingredients, please visit www.cosmeticsinfo.org."

www.burtsbees.com

www.clinique.com

http://www.californiababy.com/

▲ 1-866-288-3330

▲ Coppertone is in the process of testing all their products and updating the website to include gluten-free information. They say all their product are gluten-free.

https://dakotafree.com/Category.asp?Category_Id=5

www.ecologicalskin.com (dedicated facility)

ALWAYS READ INGREDIENTS LABELS!!!

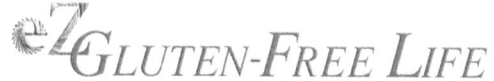

SUNSCREEN PRODUCTS	GF	VARIABLES
Hawaiian Tropic		Undetermined
Kissmyface:		
		READ
Cell Mate Facial Crème & Sunscreen	GF	
After Sun Aloe Soother	GF	
Instant Sunless Tanner	GF	
Sport Spray SPF 50	GF	
Sun Spray (Lotion SPF 30, Oil SPF 30)	GF	
Sun Swat SPF 15	GF	
Maui Babe		Undetermined
Neutrogena		Undetermined
Panama Jack		Undetermined
Shiseido	GF	
Sunology		Undetermined

VERIFIED 2013

COMPANY INFORMATION

▲ "We understand your concern about ensuring the products you are using do not contain gluten. With regard to our line of sun care products, although we do not use wheat protein or wheat derived oils in our product formulations, we cannot certify that our facilities are gluten free. In addition, the plant origin of some ingredients may vary, making Gluten Free Certification difficult. We regret we are not able to suggest a product that meets your needs at this time. For specific information on this ingredient as well as other sun care and cosmetic product ingredients, please visit www.cosmeticsinfo.org."

www.kissmyface.com
All other sunscreen may contain gluten.

http://www.mauibabe.com/
Line too extensive to give details- email about specific products
www.panamajack.com
www.shisiedo.com
www.sunology.com

ALWAYS READ INGREDIENTS LABELS!!!

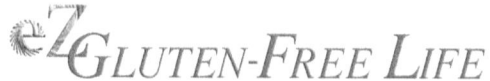

References used in this Personal Care Products Handbook:

In addition to the websites under "Company Information" and email correspondences, the below references were used while creating this reference guide.

1. Editors of Living Without.com. "So You Just Been Diagnosed with Celiac Disease...".

2. Living Without.com. August 3, 2011.

3. Green, Peter H.R. MD and Jones, Rory. Celiac Disease, A Hidden Epidemic. New York: Morrow, 2010.

4. Gluten free Delight Magazine, Copyright 2011. http://delightglutenfree.com/petergreen Matison, Mara Dr. & Matison Dainis. Cecelia's Marketplace. "Gluten-Free Grocery Shopping" Guide. Kal-Haven Publishing. Kalamazoo, MI. 2012.

5. Ratner, Amy. "Should I Worry About...Gluten in dental products." GlutenFree Living. Number 2 2011. 40,41 & 49.

6. "The CSA Gluten-Free Product Listing, 14th Edition". Celiac Sprue Association. Omaha, NE. 2010

7. http://www.celiac.com/articles/181/1/Safe-Gluten-Free-Food-List-Safe-Ingredients/Page1.html

8. http://www.celiac.org/index.php?option=com_content&view=article&id=44&Itemid=69

9. http://glutenfreedrugs.com

10. http://www.glutenfreefox.com/about.html

11. http://www.glutenfreefoodsearch.com/index.php/do-you-have-gluten-in-your-toothpaste

12. ftp://ftp.fao.org/docrep/fao/009/y5553e/y5553e01.pdf

13. http://www.gfco.org/

14. http://www.gluten.net/Quick%20Start%2006-2011.pdf

15. http://www.naturallydahling.com/Food_Allergies.html

16. Sally Hansen email

17. Boyd, Christine. "Gluten Attack: Ataxia Is gluten attacking your brain?" *Living Without Magazine.* Feb/Mar 2011 Issue. Page 4

18. Kharrazian, Datis DHSc, DC, MS. MNeuroSci. "Why Do I Still Have Thyroid Symptoms? When My Lab Results Are Normal." Elephant Printing LLC; 1 edition. February 2, 2010

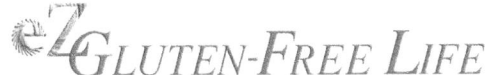

eZ GLUTEN-FREE LIFE

Acknowledgements

When you see the name of an author on the book it is only telling part of the story. Behind every author is a host of friends, family, and professionals who have given of themselves so that the author could write this book. It takes a community which inspires, encourages, guides, educates and loves the author through the process.

Dr. Cynthia Costa, thank you for my renewed health and your guidance. I remember the day Dr. Costa diagnosed me with Hashimoto's. She came into the office and leaned against the door frame. "You may never be able to eat certain foods ever again", she quietly stated as if this were a life sentence. I thought, "If that is all I have to do then bring it on." And bring it on she did. The diagnosis and eliminating gluten, dairy, soy and other foods not only improved my quality of life dramatically, it also ignited a passion in me for learning everything I could about gluten, living gluten-free, and helping others in the process. Thank you for suggesting that I become a gluten-free consultant and asking me whether or not there is gluten in numerous products. I am so grateful that Dr. Costa is my doctor, business associate, and friend.

Wendy Meg Siegel's existence defines my word for gratitude. She is my dearest and longest friend. Thank you for always being there for me. Thank you for believing in me, even when I did not believe in myself. Thank you for all your love and continued support. Thank you for your time; I know how precious it is.

My brother, Michael, is a true miracle in this journey I have been on. He is the graphic artist who designed my logo, titles of my companies, and created the blueprint for my handbooks. I cannot begin to adequately describe the endless hours he has spent helping me develop this business. He has given of his time, his talent, and his love to take my visions and make them a reality. I will be forever grateful.

My dear husband, Richard, is my rock. He loves me unconditionally, he believes in me completely, and he is always there for me.

My daughter Alexandria's birth showed me dreams do come true. She continues to inspire me every day.

I love you all!

NOTES:

NOTES:

NOTES:

NOTES:

www.ingramcontent.com/pod-product-compliance
Lightning Source LLC
Chambersburg PA
CBHW060419290526
45791CB00002B/817